SKINNY & FIT BUT NEVER HUNGRY A BIT:

YOUR PLANTASTIC GUIDE TO HEALTH, FITNESS AND THE BODY OF YOUR DREAMS

By Dr. Suzanne R. Foxx, PT, DPT

Skinny & Fit But Never Hungry A Bit; Your Plantastic Guide to Health, Fitness and the Body of Your Dreams

Cover Design by Sherri Suvarna

Front Cover Photograph by Frances Bright

TABLE OF CONTENTS:

Dedication

To my husband Dillon, and my son's Nic and Ryan, thank you for your support during the writing of this book. Without the technological support of my son, Nic, I would never have been able to complete this book.

To my twin sister and BFF, Frances Bright, and my son Nic's beautiful girlfriend, Erica Keeton, and the always helpful and kind Ed Szupel, thank you so very much for proofreading this book and for all of your helpful suggestions.

To my mother who is always cooking and my father who enjoys this so much.

And to all of my patients who have listened to my words, followed my example and my advice and as a result have changed their lives, thank you for allowing me to be a part of your healing journey.

WARNING

This book is intended for educational and entertainment purposes only and is not intended as a substitute for medical advice from a health care professional or physician. A physician should always be consulted if a person is on medication or if a person has any signs or symptoms that may require diagnosis or medical attention. You should always consult with a knowledgeable physician or other health care practitioner if you have questions or concerns about your health.

Introduction

"Healthy Foods"

Salad = 100 calories per pound

Vegetables = 200 calories per pound

Fruits = 300 calories per pound

Starches (potatoes, rice, beans) = 500 calories per pound

Nuts and seeds = 2,000-2,500 calories per pound

"Popular Foods"

Meat = 1,600 calories per pound

Cheese = 1,700 calories per pound

White Flour = 1,800 calories per pound

Sugar = 1,800 calories per pound

Chocolate = 1,800 calories per pound

Potato chips/fries = 2,500 calories per pound

Ice Cream = 3,000 calories per pound

Oil (pure fat) = 4,000 calories per pound

Hmmm…I wonder why there is an obesity epidemic in America…?

Preface

The evidence that something was going wrong with America's health was clear back in the year 1977. It was so crystal clear that Senator George McGovern of Massachusetts tried his best in order to promote a healthier diet style in order to prevent disease among the American people. This is what he said about the subject at that time:

"There is a great deal of evidence and it continues to accumulate, which strongly implicates, and in some instances proves, that the major cause of death and disability in the United States are related to the diet we eat. I include coronary artery disease, which accounts for nearly half the deaths in the United States, several of the most important forms of cancer, hypertension, diabetes and obesity as well as other chronic diseases. As a nation we have come to believe that medicine and medical technology can solve our major health problems. The role of such important factors as diet in cancer and heart disease has long been obscured by the emphasis on the conquest of these diseases through the miracles of modern medicine. Treatment, not prevention, has been the order of the day. The problems can never be solved merely by more and more medical care. The question to be asked is not why should we change our diet, but why not? What are the risks associated with less meat, less fat, less saturated fat, less cholesterol, less sugar, less salt and more fruits, vegetables, unsaturated fat and cereal products- especially whole grain cereals? There are none that can be identified and important benefits can be expected. Ischemic heart disease, cancer, diabetes and hypertension are the diseases that kill us. They are epidemic in our population. We cannot afford to temporize.

We have an obligation to inform the public of the current state of knowledge and to assist the public in making the correct food choices. To do less is to avoid our responsibility."

This was the view of the government of the United States for a few short months back in 1977. Unfortunately, it was quickly pointed out by the livestock industry that this recommendation would likely hurt their businesses and as a result the government's dietary recommendations were changed to help protect that industry. Taking the business needs of an industry into consideration when designing the health and nutrition recommendations for the average American citizen was a colossal step backward for our country, and things have only grown worse, much worse, since that time.

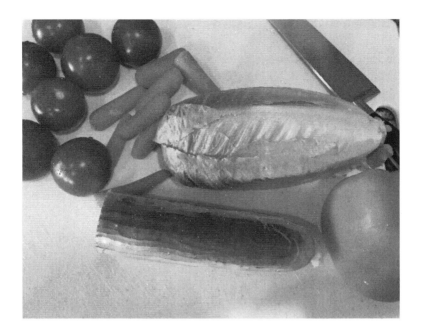

Chapter 1: The Problem

Defining the Obesity Epidemic and Explaining the Need For Change

Most people overeat to "fill up" the void caused by a complete lack of essential vitamins and minerals due to a diet high in processed junk food, salt and sugar. The truth is that although they are "overfed" they are actually undernourished.

Whether you believe in the evolutionary theory or not, of all the animals here on the planet Earth, human beings genetically most closely resemble primates, especially the great apes, and particularly chimpanzees and orangutans. We have hands with opposable thumbs (the better to pick fruit off of trees) and we have large flat molars in substantial quantities in our jaws, to crush and grind plant materials. Our teeth move in a side to side motion, to better grind the food we eat. The saliva in our mouths contains sufficient quantities of an enzyme called amylase that begins breaking down carbohydrates upon ingestion, rather than waiting for the stomach to start the process, as carnivores primarily do. We cannot manufacture Vitamin C inside of our bodies like most other animals can, and thus must obtain it from our diets, just like other primates. Did you know that most other mammals, especially the carnivorous ones, can make their own Vitamin C?

If you are a religious person, you likely believe that we were made in God's image. My belief is that we were made in God's image from materials available here on the earth. We were made in God's image based on a primate "chassis". Unlike the great apes, we, as humans, have long, strong legs for running. Our running ability is amazing and separates us from most other animals. We may not be the fastest runners in the world, but we certainly have the most endurance. We can even run far enough and long enough to run down wild game because of our unique ability to sweat through our skin. Other animals, including horses and cheetahs, must stop to pant and catch their breath after short bursts of sprinting. Human beings are uniquely able to keep on running, mile after mile. With that being said, the animal foods we eat, if we choose to eat them, are supposed to be in small quantities and obtained only after heroically long runs and quite a lot of physical labor (clubbing it to death, cutting it in strips, building a fire, cooking it and then eating it).

Not many human beings run or exercise like this anymore, even if they participate in extreme sports such as the fitness program Cross Fit, or regularly participate in doing the P90X workout or train and prepare for long distance runs like 5k's, 10k's, half marathon, marathons and even longer distance running.

When hunting activities took place among our ancient ancestors, it was likely done a few times a year as a group effort and bonding experience and was certainly not an everyday activity. I think most of the hunting and gathering that was done amounted to mostly gathering. Hunting, by its nature, has a significant element of danger, and the chance that the hunters would come back empty handed, or even worse, injured or killed, was high. As long as ancient people could also gather, there was enough food for everyone, at least those who survived long enough to reproduce. The people who survived from this time in history are the ones we have all descended from.

Assuming that evolutionary theory has its place, and that we resemble the great apes, with the exception of our ability to run, consider what you would feed a large ape or chimpanzee that came to your house to eat. Would you jolt him awake with a shot or two of caffeine mixed with cream and sugar when he wakes up every morning? For breakfast, would you feed him cereal splashed with the milk of a cow or sugar and fat laden doughnuts? For lunch, would you feed him pizza topped with pepperoni slices and extra cheese and with the crust stuffed with even more cheese with chicken wings in special hot sauce on the side? For supper, would you feed him a great big bowl of spaghetti and meat balls with double cheese garlic bread and ice cream for dessert? How about a pork chop with mashed potatoes smothered in gravy and chocolate pie a la mode for dessert? What would happen to your monkey friend if you fed him this way night after night and day after day? Imagine him drinking carbonated, highly sweetened cola with bubbles several times a day. What if we indulged him with energy shots of caffeine and extra candy and potato chips sprinkled in throughout the day? Imagine him drinking two to three glasses of wine every evening. Imagine him sipping several beers with his friends on a regular basis.

The evidence of what your poor monkey friend would look like can be seen all around you. He would be fat, and if he was over thirty years old, he would also be sick. He would be sick enough to require daily medication and regular veterinary care. The medication prescribed to him by his well-meaning veterinarian would cause side effects and wouldn't do anything to really solve his problems. The medication would just mask and manage the symptoms for a while. Even if this monkey exercised on a regular basis, he would still be fat. He would still be fat and he would still be sick. No amount of exercise can ever replace a good diet.

As a young monkey, with just the right combination of genes, his body may have better coping mechanisms because he would naturally be more active. He may be able to remain strong and healthy on the diet plan above, but if you continued to feed him this way for several years, your monkey has a seventy to eighty percent chance of becoming fat. He has a thirty percent chance of becoming obese.

With all of the excess weight he would likely experience the onset of disease processes like hypertension, high cholesterol, atherosclerosis, heart disease, Type II diabetes and even many forms of cancer. His weight bearing joints would be overburdened by the excess weight and he would likely have pain and dysfunction in them, especially his knees. Your monkey's vet bills would mount to thousands of dollars per year as he came down with every chronic disease that has a name. He would require shovels full of pills every day just to keep his miserable carcass around for several more years.

If he is a good friend of yours, you would probably wonder why he is so sick and how this could have been prevented, all while making him another ham, cheese and mayonnaise sandwich on white bread, served with his favorite highly salted potato chips and with his favorite soda to drink. If you were really worried about him, you might make him eat cartons of yogurt and drink fruit juice instead of soda. These supposed "health foods" would have little effect on his health and his veterinary care bills would continue to rise.

Look around you. I hardly need to explain that the great nation of the United States of America is the home of the fat and the free. Everywhere you look in America you can see people who are struggling with excess body weight. If you walk down the street, through a store, or go to a restaurant and look around, most of the people that you see will be overweight and many of them will be obese.

The statistics are staggering. Seventy percent of Americans are overweight and thirty percent of them are heavy enough to be considered obese. A person is considered to be obese if their body mass index, or BMI, is above thirty. BMI can be calculated with this complicated mathematical formula.

BMI = {Weight in pounds / Height (Inches)x Height (Inches)} x 703

Based on this formula, a person of either gender who is 5 feet, 6 inches tall should weigh between 115 and 155 pounds. This same person is considered to be overweight if they weigh between 156 pounds and 185 pounds. If they weigh 186 pounds or more they are then considered to be obese using the BMI calculation. A normal BMI falls between 18.5 and 24.9. A person is overweight if their BMI falls between 25.0 and 29.9. A person is considered obese if their BMI is above 30.0.

Body mass index does have its flaws as it only takes into account height and weight and not body composition. For the most part, it is pretty accurate in diagnosing who is, and who is not overweight. In fact many experts feel that it is all too lenient in determining who is overweight, as a female that is 5 feet 6 inches tall and weighs 155 pounds is, in all likelihood, overweight, but her BMI will still fall within the normal range. The only people who really have a high BMI but are incredibly fit are usually athletes in very good shape who have minimal body fat and a great deal of muscle mass because muscle weighs more than fat. So, if you do not work out regularly, and you do not eat healthfully, and if your waist is larger than your chest, and you have a BMI that is above 25, then you are overweight.

Here, in the United States, even the children and the household pets are struggling with excessive weight. The children, of course, eat what their parent's do, so this could account for their weight problems, if we are to assume the problem is both genetic and related to diet. However, that does not explain why the pets are overweight. What about the pets? How come our pets are so fat? If the problem is poor genes, then how come our pets are fat too? As much as we love our pets, they are not genetically related to us, and yet they, too, are fat and often, unfortunately, obese. They often suffer many of the same health problems that plague the rest of us. Could it be that they, too, are also malnourished from eating the wrong things?

Everyone proclaims to want to be of normal weight, feel good and look great in their clothes. Personally, I do not know anyone, nor have I ever met anyone, who says that they would like to be overweight or obese. There are some people who proclaim to want to have "some meat on their bones", but even they would like to be curvy, or well muscled, and not obese. Instead I have spent a great deal of time with people who say they would do anything and they have tried everything to lose excess weight and that it is just not possible for them.

I know that when a person is overweight, being of normal weight seems like an impossible goal to achieve. Everyone has heard of a solution that promises to aid them in their weight loss journey. Most people can follow a diet plan for a few weeks, and sometimes, with heroic effort, even for a few months, but sticking with it for a lifetime just seems like an impossible task. Realistically there is just too much temptation everywhere you go and nobody can stand to deprive themselves in a world where food is plentiful and so easily attainable, especially when their stomachs are growling.

As Americans, we constantly hear about how our country spends more on health care than any other country in the world, and yet we are still in miserable physical condition as one of the fattest and unhealthiest nations. The number one killer of Americans is heart disease, a disease brought on by years of poor nutrition and overindulgence in all of the wrong things. Is it just inevitable that so many of us must die from this disease?

Once diagnosed, heart disease is usually managed for many years with medications, invasive tests and procedures and with ever increasing rates of disability, until nothing else can be done and the inevitable deadly heart attack or stroke occurs.

You might find yourself wondering what can be done about this. There is so much conflicting information about nutrition and how to become healthy and what you are and aren't supposed to do to get there. All of this information can be very confusing. When it comes to nutrition and exercise information there are a staggering number of different sources available ranging from celebrities and trainers, the internet, TV and even our neighbors and coworkers.

There are the high protein camps with the very low and no carbohydrate diet plans following the Adkins train of thought. There are the no fruit police and the pill, shake and supplement pushers. There are the special device salespeople who hawk their versions of slimming clothing that can be worn and special exercise equipment that you can buy. Diet plans that are often mentioned include carb counting, purple mangosteen pills and drinks, green coffee extracts, the latest fruit extract, green tea, Chinese tea, experimental medications, gastric bypass surgery and lap banding. There are shakes, bars, protein mixes and smoothies. All of these plans promise fast and easy weight loss. And for some reason they all sound like snake oil at best with a cost of $129.95 or more on an automatic credit card draft every month, tied, of course, to an active bank account that happens to belong to you!

All of these weight loss ideas come with their own theories and different promises, but the fact is that most do not actually work for most people, if they work at all. This is especially true for long term results, which is what most people would like to achieve. Americans spend twenty billion dollars, that is billion, with a B, on weight loss aids every year. If even one of them worked as promised, then America's obesity problem would be solved. At least one of these ridiculous ideas would have taken hold and stuck and there would be a serious turn around to our countries current trend of becoming fatter and sicker every year. I once heard that if you go to the drug store and there are multiple "so called" solutions to the problem that you are experiencing, then the likely truth is that there is no real agreed upon method for fixing the problem, just a lot of stuff that works a little bit. Nothing seems to REALLY work. The pills, the carb counting, the devices, they just don't work, or they work a little tiny bit for a very short period of time. People can torture themselves and do these things for short periods of time, but it is very likely that they cannot keep this up forever. How in the world did this country end up like this?

This problem, in which nearly every adult over the age of thirty is overweight and /or taking medications for chronic health conditions, seems to be a fairly new phenomenon.

I grew up in the 1970's on an Air Force base in Illinois. From there, my family moved to Minnesota and then overseas to Germany. I remember in the seventies that there were overweight people here and there but they weren't EVERYWHERE! They existed, but they did not constitute seventy percent of the adult population! There were more like one or two chubby kids in the neighborhood. Somewhere between ten and twenty percent of the adults were overweight and maybe, once in a while, there would be a really large, obese person, who could only wear a mu-mu or very large workout pants, as there were no clothes made that were large enough to fit them. That kind of obesity was rare. So what is going on now? How come now there are so many overweight people in this country? How did this happen? What has changed between then and now?

In the 1970's, when I was a child, there was only one overweight child in the whole grade. Sadly enough today if you walk into an elementary school there are at least six or more overweight children in each classroom. The parents and caretakers of these children are often in complete denial about the situation and the fact that they are likely major contributors to the problem. They will tell you that they feed the child a healthy diet and that he/she gets plenty of exercise. They often won't allow the child to eat candy publicly. They sign this child up for two or three sports related activities with their ensuing practice sessions and then spend huge amounts of time driving this child to all of the necessary events every evening and on the weekends. Of course with all of these activities and all of this driving around in the evenings and on weekends there is no time for healthy food preparation. But there is also no need for food preparation when there is a fat, I mean fast food restaurant on every corner that promises to take care of this boring chore quickly and easily.

Just thinking about why this child has a weight problem doesn't even seem to make sense. Who is to blame? Should we blame this on the schools? Is it the fault of the television? Is it the video games? Is this problem all caused by all of the easily purchased and consumed cheap junk food items available at fast food restaurants? All of these things mentioned here are ultimately controlled by the parents of this child. Realistically this has to be the fault of the parents and the caregivers of the child. Children do not buy groceries. Children do not make decisions about where and what to eat. Children can only complain about their choices and beg their parents for certain items, but they ultimately make no purchases of their own. Most of the time, when a child is overweight or obese, their parents are too. In most of these situations, all that the parents need to do to find the source of their child's weight problem is to look into the mirror and see who is helping to perpetuate this insanity.

What is even more amazing to me is how all of this has taken place over the last twenty to thirty years. Childhood obesity used to be rare and it is now commonplace. Advertisements are now starting to include overweight and obese children in the images of children portrayed on their products as this becomes the new normal and the advertisers want everyone to feel included in the marketing of their products.

There are so many overweight people everywhere that you look. Nobody wants to be overweight. If you ask each of these individuals they will all tell you that they eat a healthy diet and that they exercise, maybe not regularly, but they have tried everything to lose excess weight and are just unable. Some of these people will tell you that they believe that they have faulty genes, a slow intestinal process, and a slow metabolism or even that they are genetically "big boned" and naturally large in size. They may also tell you how in the not so distant past they ran for miles and were able to perform amazing athletic feats. They will tell you how even though they are larger than they should be, they are healthy. In fact, they will insist on stating that they are healthy.

But truthfully, healthy people are not overweight just like genetics does not account for overweight pets. There is a logical cause to this problem and thus a logical solution to this problem. The good news is that if the problem is our fault, then we are in control of it and we can fix it. If we are the cause of the problem, then we are also the solution. It is not out of our control, it is very much within our control.

I have also suffered from being heavier than I would like to be. I have spent years fighting the battle of an excess five to twenty pounds depending on the year and circumstances. Every few years I would begin to notice a bit of a weight problem. My clothes would start to get tight. I would notice a muffin top forming around my midsection and pooling out over the top of my pants and a general widening of my hips. I would then try to look for a special diet that I would follow for a few months to get back on track. Calorie restriction diets worked well when I was in my twenties and early thirties. But the number of allowed calories just kept getting smaller and smaller for the same results. After a while I was down to eating less than 1200 calories a day, starving, irritable and cold all of the time, and still unable to lose the excess weight. The very last time I tried a calorie restriction diet, I ate a diet of 1200 calories per day for three months and went from 143 pounds to 138 pounds while running on a treadmill for between fifteen and twenty miles a week. I was completely miserable. All of my efforts gave me very little results. The scale barely changed and I felt completely discouraged and like a complete failure.

Below I have included a few of the sample menus from my last restricted calorie diet routine. As you read through the menu plan, I am sure you will find that you, too, have tried a similar plan in the past.

Monday

7 -11 French Vanilla Cappuccino   200

Little Caesar's Cheese Pizza – 3 slices   360

5 Girl Scout Samoa Cookies   350

Frozen Asparagus Spears   45

Vanilla Yogurt Cup 180

Total Calories for the Day: 1035

Tuesday

7 -11 French Vanilla Cappuccino   200

Banana   100

Lays Potato Chips   160

Slice of Lemon Loaf Cake   200

Amy's Enchilada Frozen Entrée   240

Total Calories for the Day: 900

Wednesday

7 -11 French Vanilla Cappuccino   200

2 Fried Eggs   140

Butter used to fry eggs   100

Wendy's Fish Sandwich – No tartar sauce   450

Granola Bar   170

Blueberry Yogurt Cup   120

Total Calories for the Day: 1180

Thursday

½ Brownie   100

7 -11 French Vanilla Cappuccino   200

Macaroni and Cheese from KFC   370

Cheese Nips Crackers snack pack   210

Amy's Enchilada's 240

Kozy Shack Rice Pudding Cup150

Total Calories for the Day: 1295

Friday

Banana   100

7 -11 French Vanilla Cappuccino   200

Cheese Pizza 2 slices   500

Welch's Fruit Snacks   80

Tomato cut into slices with salt and pepper x 2   44

Popcorn 3.5 ounces at cirque de soliel   250

Snow cone at cirque de soliel 80

Total Calories for the Day: 1254

Saturday

2 Fried Eggs   140

Butter used to fry eggs   100

2 Slices of Honey Wheat Toast   140

Butter on the Toast 100

Orange Juice   150

7 -11 French Vanilla Cappuccino   200

Banana   100

Vegetarian Bean Burrito 250

Total Calories for the Day 1180

Sunday

Yogurt Cup   120

Diet Dr. Pepper   0

Chili's Black Bean Burger with Bun, Cheese slice, ketchup,

Tomato and Lettuce   650

7 -11 French Vanilla Cappuccino   200

Mashed Potatoes   250

Total Calories for the Day 1220

This menu plan accurately reflects my life as I am very busy and not very good at planning my meals in advance. This was what I could easily eat without having to go to a lot of trouble. I know that this is what other people eat too. Like most American's, I tend to be a picky eater. I never have been much of a cook but I only like to eat things that taste pretty good. The French Vanilla Cappuccino from 7 –Eleven was my salvation during my calorie restricting dieting days. It helped me to feel warm and comfortable for the short time while I drank it and made the rest of these miserable weeks and months possible. Everyone deserves a treat, right? My life is very busy and I feel rushed most of the time but I could savor this beverage and it really did make me feel better. It warmed my cold, flaking skin and hands and helped me feel human despite the pitiful amount of food I was otherwise "allowed" to eat. Let me explain the flaking skin.

For some reason, in my twenties, I had developed a skin condition all over my head and neck which resembled psoriasis and consisted of oily and painful skin flaking. I had seen several physicians who had diagnosed the rash as just a really bad case of common dandruff. I was advised to use a strong prescription strength shampoo and to apply a steroid cream. The shampoo left my hair feeling dry and brittle. The shine was gone from my hair and it was very frizzy. The cream was smelly and made my hair look greasy and flat. These medications did help to clear the condition up, but only by about thirty percent. They never cleared the condition completely. I am embarrassed to admit that I had such a condition, but I have learned that everyone has things that they have to deal with. This skin condition seemed to be one of those problems for me.

At around the same time that the skin on my head began to itch and flake, I was also getting ill frequently, suffering from at least six upper respiratory infections from cold viruses a year with laryngitis every winter that would typically last from February to April. This had been going on for about seven years in a row. I also had frequent headache pain and a general aching in my joints besides the constant cold I felt from a general lack of calories and very likely anemia as well.

As a practicing medical professional, a physical therapist, I felt that I was just getting older and that this must be how it feels and what happens to the aging body, a feeling that I am sure most people over thirty years old can relate to. I had to exert a tremendous amount of self-control to keep from eating more than my regimented 1200 - 1500 calories per day and there were several days where I was completely finished eating by three o'clock in the afternoon. I had to maintain my health with exercise so I would try to run or walk on a treadmill at home several nights per week but often, at the end of the day, I was so hungry and so exhausted that admittedly this was very difficult to do. Often I felt like I would be better off holding my eyelids open with toothpicks at the end of the day.

At the same time, I thought to myself, that this seemed completely insane and that there had to be a better way. People cannot live like this! It just couldn't be right that people are expected to maintain such high levels of self-control that they are completely miserable most of the time. Who wouldn't need a little comforting in the form of food with all of the skin itching, fatigue, headaches and aching joint pain?

I had already tried taking multivitamins intermittently to try and help on several previous occasions and frankly, the scientific journal articles available on the subject of vitamin supplementation were and still remain really scary. All of the scientific literature seemed to point to an excessive intake of supplemental vitamins as a possible cause of increased cancer risk in certain populations and with certain vitamin supplements. These certain vitamin supplements happened to be any and all of the ones that had actually been researched heavily! This is, and continues to be alarming. It seems like every time a vitamin supplement is researched using the gold standard of testing, which is a double blind study, the results are always an increased cancer incidence in the experimental group; the one that has been receiving the excessive amount of whatever vitamin is being studied. This was not the case with actual foods, however, just vitamins derived from those foods. Living in the United States and eating a traditional or standard American Diet, I always felt that taking vitamins and minerals was unnecessary anyway. As a health care professional I had learned during my training that most people, if they eat a variety of foods and get enough calories to eat ,very likely do not need to take any supplements.From what I remembered from health classes, both in high school and college, as well as generally available articles in magazines and newspapers, is that for the most part, none of us need to worry about a lack of any specific nutrients that would require supplementation. This is especially true in a country that is as affluent and powerful as the United States. The general consensus seems to be that physician's very rarely see a person who is suffering from a real vitamin or mineral deficiency here in the United States because of the amazing availability and variety of foods in this country and the way that so many of the typical foods eaten by Americans are fortified with the essential and necessary nutrients.

Vitamin and mineral deficiencies are usually only seen in third world countries or in those individuals that for some reason or another are eating a very unnatural and restrictive diet. I felt that I was able to obtain plenty of nutrients on the standard American diet and that supplementation of any kind was an unnecessary bandage. This is what I was taught and what I firmly believed and still believe to this day.

I truly feel that most supplements are not likely necessary and may even be harmful. All these supplements do is make expensive urine but are otherwise completely unnecessary with one exception, Vitamin B12 and possibly vitamin D, depending on what part of the country you live in and what season it happens to be.

Most human beings over the age of fifty years old will not be able to absorb Vitamin B12 as readily as they once were able to and most people older than fifty will require supplementation of Vitamin B12, no matter what kind of diet that they eat.

Vegan diets are also lacking in Vitamin B12. Here is the reason why. Vitamin B12 is absolutely essential for many functions in the body. It is made by bacteria. Meat products and animal derived foods all contain varying amounts of vitamin B12 because of the bacteria on the meat and in the animal products. The meat does not make the Vitamin B12, rather it is grown by bacteria that live on and in the meat. When people ingest this bacteria laden meat, they naturally eat the bacteria and obtain Vitamin B12 in this way. Well water is another source of naturally occurring B12 in the human diet. Because human beings no longer drink untreated well water (which again, contains bacteria) and because we wash the dirt and bacteria off of our fruits and vegetables before we eat them, we cannot count on obtaining enough Vitamin B12 by eating fruit and vegetables alone.

As a result, we need to take Vitamin B12 once or twice a week while eating a vegan diet or near vegan diet. All people over fifty years old should take this important vitamin regardless of their diet. It is easily supplemented, not expensive and one bottle will last you a very long time.

Vitamin D is the other Vitamin that may need to be supplemented. Many foods are fortified with Vitamin D to be sure that the body is able to obtain enough. Vitamin D does not occur naturally in any food item but instead is a hormone made by our bodies when our skin is exposed to sunlight. Because of the tilt of the earth and the places that we live, the clothes that we wear and the sunscreen that we use, we may not have enough sun exposure to allow our bodies to make adequate amounts of vitamin D with sun exposure alone. Vitamin D is necessary for strong bones. I do not supplement my diet with any other vitamins other than these two vitamins, B12 and D. I do not believe that it is necessary for human beings eating a truly healthy diet to take any other kinds of vitamins and I do not advocate that they do so. I think that the scientific evidence on the subject seems pretty clear that breaking one vitamin out of its natural packaging and sending it into the body can actually be more harmful than beneficial.

Another common misconception is that people need to concentrate on their food, and eat without any type of distractions, in order to be of a healthy weight. Right before Thanksgiving one year, I retrieved the newspaper from my driveway and I turned to an article written by a diet expert that was intended to help people control the amount of weight that they would inevitably gain over the upcoming holiday season. The article stated that the average American would pack on about eight extra pounds over Thanksgiving, Christmas and New Year's. The article was filled with advice about how to keep off this inevitable weight gain.

The supposed helpful suggestions included ideas such as to chew every mouthful of food at least twenty times, don't multitask while you eat but instead concentrate on smelling and tasting each bite of food, as well as only eating the foods that you really enjoy. It was also suggested that a person eat only one serving of each truly favorite food. Another absurd suggestion offered by this article was that each individual should write a list of the reasons that they wanted to be thin and to read the list every morning and throughout the day if they were feeling like they may start overeating.

The article actually mentioned a class that this diet expert was teaching in which the participants, mostly middle aged overweight females, were to take a nutrition bar, break it up in small pieces and smell and feel each morsel prior to placing it into their mouths to eat it. This exercise was to help them savor and appreciate each bite and to be "in the moment...." enjoying each tiny bite.

As I read this article all I could think about was how demeaning all of this advice is. It is absolutely ridiculous to have grown adults sitting around sniffing a nutrition bar, which probably doesn't even taste good, and hoping that they will have enough self-control and that with enough effort they will eat it slowly and carefully, chewing each bite twenty times, paying close attention to each sensation they experienced, and tell themselves that they would be thin and beautiful if they were only able to eat all of their food in this manner. I don't know about you but this does not sound like a great way to enjoy the holidays, does it?

I think it is a lot easier to be thin and beautiful when you are full and not feeling deprived of anything. A lack of self-control cannot possibly be to blame for the enormous obesity problem that we have in our country today. Americans are some of the hardest working people in the entire world, taking the fewest holidays and working much more than many other civilized societies.

As Americans, when we have a goal in mind, we are unstoppable and rarely get side-tracked. There is just no way that an entire country can lack self-control. If seventy percent of us had cancerous tumors on our faces or spontaneously developed a crippling disease at the age of twenty, there would definitely be a reason for it and you can be sure that the government would pump billions of our tax dollars into figuring out what it was and how to fix it. Why this is not happening with the obesity epidemic says a lot about our nation's priorities.

Clearly, there is a reason for America's obesity problem. It is definitely a fairly new phenomenon. Obviously, there is something wrong. And the problem is not a lack of self-control. It has been drilled into all of us over and over again that taking in too many calories of ANY kind leads to weight gain and obesity.

I now firmly disagree with this principle. After my personal journey and with my intensive studying and investigation of this matter, I have discovered that it is WHAT we eat rather than how much of it that we eat that determines our weight, our general health and our physical condition. It would be amazing if the health of this nation could be restored with something as simple as good nutrition. Wouldn't it be staggering to suggest that American's, who are some of the richest people in the world, are actually the ones that are suffering from malnutrition?

I am now convinced that nearly everyone in the United States who has been eating the standard traditional American Diet is actually suffering from malnutrition and a lack of significant micronutrients and phytochemicals in their diet. As a result of this lack of micronutrients, the body is thrown into a state of constant craving where the message sent to the brain by the digestive system is to keep on eating in order to provide enough substance to possibly attain these very necessary micronutrients. Like mining for gold by sifting through tons of sand on a beach, the body's digestive system demands huge amounts of food in order to find the very small amounts of micronutrients available in their natural packages so that they can be easily taken up and utilized by the body.

The real problem is that there is absolutely no actual nutritional value in most of the foods that are regularly eaten by Americans. This has nothing to do with soil depletion or the use of organic versus conventionally grown produce. It comes down to a significant LACK of fruits, vegetables, beans, nuts and seeds, also known as PRODUCE, in the typical American's diet.

Most American's simply do not eat enough produce. In fact, on a daily basis, most Americans really don't eat any produce at all. None. Zilch. Nada. Nothing. I believe that this serious lack of produce consumption is responsible for most of the diseases and pathological processes that are common to American's and those in other westernized nations. This complete lack of produce consumption is responsible for the obesity epidemic and the ensuing diabetes and hypertension epidemics.

A lack of produce in the diet has been linked to many different kinds of cancer and is responsible for most of the cases of heart disease. As highly complex primates, the human body is constantly craving nutritious foods and Americans keep eating junk in an attempt to stop the craving, which does nothing to meet the actual needs of the body. Because the actual nutritional needs have not been met, the digestive system signals the brain which tells the person to consume even more food, which again contains nothing of actual nutritional value and so the cycle continues.

After reading this book and educating yourself on just how easy and satisfying it can be to eat a proper diet, I have no doubt that you will want to implement this plan and regain your health as well as control of your body weight. If you choose not to do this, then you have to accept the truth that you simply don't WANT to be thin and healthy.

Just like a smoker has to accept the fact that they really do not want to stop smoking, eating junk all day, every day is something that you have to really want to stop doing. In order to quit eating junk or to quit smoking, you have to truly want to stop it. The truth is that just a few days without cigarettes and a few days without junk food will change everything, from your outlook to your priorities and your future plans and this will make these damaging, addictive behaviors unnecessary. Taking the steps to get on top of bad, unhealthy habits builds confidence and strength in ways that nothing else can. This is easy but it is different and you will simply have to DO IT.

A typical excuse for not being able to eat properly is that it is too hard or expensive or involves too much preparation or that you simply cannot tolerate being hungry all of the time. Other common excuses are that you are simply too busy and you don't want to think so much about what you are going to eat. You have so many other things going on that you simply have no time to add one more thing to your already over loaded schedule.

The good news is that this plan does not involve anything difficult at all. This plan is very easy to implement and follow and it involves absolutely no starvation or even hunger pain. If you read through this plan and find that you are just not able to do this then it is because you choose not to do it. It will not be because it is too hard or because you will be too hungry or that it is too expensive.

Wanting something and actually doing it by taking the necessary steps to accomplish a goal are two different matters. After all, seventy percent of Americans are overweight and supposedly unhappy about it. You have to ask yourself, are you really unhappy about your weight and your health, or are you just saying that you are?

I know that when I was overweight, I was REALLY unhappy about it. I was REALLY tired of all the suffering and I was willing to do whatever was necessary to become healthy and happy again. This plan is so easy and so healthful that there is no need to prepare separate meals for other members of the family and no need to feel deprived of anything. This plan is so easy that I could follow it myself.

I am a person who does not like to cook and wants to spend the minimal amount of time that is possible in a kitchen and at the grocery store. Even I followed this plan and continue to maintain it and I easily lost all of the weight that I cared to lose. This plan is so easy that even my husband lost weight and reversed his Type II diabetes, hypertension and high cholesterol by following it.

The truth is that if you do not choose to just go ahead with this plan, following it until you have reached your ideal weight, and maintaining it to maximize your health, then you are not really interested in getting thinner and healthier and you are happy with how things are right now.

This plan is for people who are really fed up and really want to change. It is for those who really need a plan that works every time for every one without exception. This plan is not too hard and it is not too radical. It is different and it will require you to change. The truth is that if you implement this plan and it does not work for you, then you really didn't do it. If you try it and it does not work then it is likely that you are lying to yourself about what you are and are not eating. If change is not something that you are interested in doing then you will not be successful with this plan. You cannot do this half way; you must do this ninety-seven percent of the time. This means it must be fully implemented three hundred and fifty five days of the year every year that you are alive to be effective. The other ten days of the year will hardly matter. The truth comes down to this one simple fact. You have to WANT to change.

NO ONE CAN MAKE YOU DO IT.

Not your spouse, not your doctor, not your parents, not your children and not your friends.

Wanting to change comes from within and you have to really want to do it.

I wanted to change so badly. I just didn't know how to get where I wanted to be without suffering and even when I chose the path of starvation and suffering, I still did not attain my goals. After long periods of research and much experimentation I have been led to this solution and this plan, which worked amazingly fast and has made be extraordinarily happy.

The truth is I wanted it so badly that I was actually willing to do the scariest thing of all and that was....to change. I WANTED to change and was willing to take the necessary steps to get the job done. I WANTED to be thin and healthy and I WANTED to feel better about myself. This WANTING made me actually DO IT and that is what you will have to do too. Nobody else can do this for you, you have to make up your mind to do it.

This plan will not be difficult or time consuming; however it will be different from what you are doing right now. You have to make up your mind right now that you will actually DO what is required. You have to WANT it badly enough that you will keep going even when and if obstacles and conflicts arise. If your work schedule changes, if your friends are angry, if your parents, siblings, children and spouse are upset about it, if you are in the process of moving, or you have young children or you are caring for a loved one that is ill, you have to persist anyway.

YOU HAVE TO MAKE UP YOUR MIND.

The obstacles will come from expected and unexpected places. Obstacles will come in the form of people judging you and placing their own insecurities on you and telling you that you are too thin, that this is ridiculous and that it is not possible to be healthy eating the way that you do. People will tell you that your children's health will suffer if you "deprive" them of traditional American staples such as pizza, fish shaped snack crackers, juice in boxes and gummy fruit flavored snacks, which are all really just junk food.

Just because you don't want to be overweight and unhealthy people will be angry with you. You have to be prepared because sometimes other people may be a little bit angry with you when you succeed in doing what they have failed at repeatedly and they will be even angrier when they see you a year later and you are still skinny and fit and they have gained all of the weight back that they had lost doing the Paleo, Wheat Belly, Adkins, Weight Watchers, Sugar Busters, or the Blood type diet. They will have gained all of the weight back and perhaps even more weight than they had lost. I see this all of the time.

Because of your success you may be excluded from social events. Your friends may not be interested in having you over as you will be there all thin and healthy and grinning from ear to ear with the results of your success and you WILL want to share it with them and they will be angry and they will not want to listen. You will want to tell them how easy it was, but they will not want to hear what you have to say. Others will not likely be happy with your success. The reason for this is because if you did it then maybe it is possible for them to do it too and the truth is that they don't want to change anything. They simply want to do nothing and they want that to be ok. Change is difficult for everyone.

These are the barriers, or walls, to your success that will be around you as you start and complete this journey.

In just a few months, you will be thin and a few months after that, you will be healthy. THIS WILL BE A HUGE CHANGE. Just keep in mind that the barriers to success are only built up to keep out the people who do not WANT success badly enough to either knock the walls down or crawl up and over the top of them or dig up under them. In the end, these figurative walls that are built to stop your success end up being erected entirely by YOU and YOU are the only one that can take them down.

Let me be perfectly clear, this plan is a matter of will power only in that YOU have to WANT to do it. You have to WANT to change. If you do not WANT it, then you will not do it and you will not be skinny, fit, healthy and beautiful. Eating this way and living this way will help you to maximize your potential and will help you on your journey to being the best person that you can be. If you do not want to do it and choose not to do it you will more than likely look like everyone else in America, overweight, bloated, popping pills for numerous chronic health conditions and complaining that nothing seems to work to help with your health and weight problems. You will continue eating your boxed junk containing meal that you simply add hamburger, tuna or chicken to or takeout pizza or Chinese food with canned green beans on the side, drinking a soda and wondering why you always feel so sick and tired and weak and are aching all over. Trips to your physician's office will not make you any better, they won't even come close. Medication alone can never make you truly well. Physician's offices and hospitals offer sick care, not well care.

So where are you mentally? Do you really want to change or are you still at the "thinking it through" stage? Change is change and by its very nature it will be difficult, but it isn't really that hard once you are mentally ready to do it. Understand that none of this will be difficult if you set your mind straight in the beginning. This plan isn't difficult when you are really ready to go. When you are really ready it will be easier because you will have CHANGED YOUR MIND.

And changing your mind is the most difficult part of the whole process.

If your mind is set and you are ready to begin a journey of real health and wellness, then continue with this book. The plan that I propose does not require suffering and starvation or unrealistic goals and expectations. It is real. It takes minimal effort but it does require a change in your mental state and attitude.

You will be required to change your mind about what is and is not real food. You will be required to obtain the majority of your daily calories from real, nutrient containing food and not "fake food." or animal products, which are nutrient poor choices. You will be required to read nutritional labels and eat "party" type foods only at real parties and on special occasions. These special occasions only occur five to ten days per year, and certainly not every day. These will be the changes that you must make.

If you are still reading then you are probably ready to find out exactly how this plan works. First and foremost, you have to decide that you really want to change. This is the most important step. Without deciding that you really want to change, you will fail.

So have you decided? Are you ready to really do it? Promise yourself that you will really give this a try and do this for at least six weeks. That is not a really long time. If you are nineteen years old, then six weeks may seem like a really long time, but really, it is just a month and a half. Isn't it amazing to think that in a month and a half your whole life could be different? Or in six weeks, if you do nothing, you could be right where you are right now. If you do nothing, then nothing will happen and the result will be just that, nothing. The reason you need a time commitment of six weeks is because change, even good and positive change, can be difficult. There will be times when you want to give up and it is important that you honor your commitment, at least for six weeks. It will not be hard, it will just be different.

I am convinced that if you try this, in six weeks you will feel so much better that you will never go back. This will become a part of your new life and you will wonder how you even lived the way that you used to. If you can commit to six weeks, then keep on reading. If not, then put this book away for a while and think about whether you really want to change or not. Maybe after you have looked in the mirror or after you come back from your scary doctor's office visit where they are suggesting all kinds of pills and procedures or after your knees give out on you as you go up the stairs or after the top button on your pants won't button anymore, you will come back to this book and this plan.

Come back to this book when you are good and fed up with how things are going and when you have decided that enough is enough and you are willing to do the hardest thing of all, which is to change.

If you are ready, let's begin...

Throughout this process, keep in mind that:

A bad attitude is like a flat tire. You can't go anywhere until you change it.

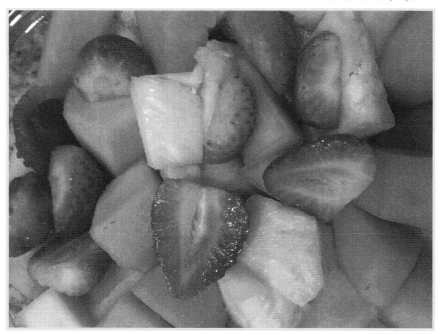

Chapter 2: Your Doctor Probably Doesn't Know Very Much About Human Nutrition:

Explaining the Role of Medical Science in Maintaining Human Health

Does your family doctor look healthy? Is he or she in good physical condition? Is he or she generally thin with good muscle tone? Does he or she exercise regularly and eat a healthy diet most of the time? Do his or her eyes look bright? Is his or her hair smooth and shiny? Is his or her skin free of blemishes and have a natural pink healthy glow?

53

Does he or she look like a person who is a great example of good physical health and condition? Does he or she look a little athletic? Like he or she could run a couple of miles, do a few pushups and sit ups and still have energy left to be a good doctor?

Physicians today are very well trained. Your doctor is likely capable of saving your life. He or she has advanced training and is capable of coming up with a treatment plan for most any pathology that you bring to his or her office. If your doctor does not have the expertise himself, he or she knows where to send you for advanced disease treatment and testing for pathological conditions. Keeping you alive is the goal of today's medical practice. Keeping you healthy and in good physical condition is entirely up to you.

You wouldn't dream of getting your haircut from someone who has a poorly maintained hairstyle. You wouldn't ask for lawn care tips from someone whose yard is full of weeds and crabgrass and is otherwise dead and brown. You wouldn't ask for the recipe of a dish that is greasy, overcooked and too salty at a pot luck picnic. It wouldn't make sense to do these things. Taking dietary and exercise advice from an overweight and unhealthy person, even if that person happens to be a well-trained physician, isn't prudent either.

Statistically, forty -two percent of male physicians and thirty two percent of female physicians are overweight.

(This information comes from the online journal Medscape's discussion of overweight physicians.) Physicians, as a rule, are doing better at managing their weight and their health than average Americans are, but many of them are fat and sick too. This doesn't mean that they can't save your life, they can and they will. It just means that they don't know enough about nutrition and exercise to maintain themselves in excellent physical condition and good health. If they don't know enough about these two topics to maintain their own body, how will they be able to help you to maintain yours?

This is not meant to be judgmental of today's often overworked and underpaid physicians. They are absolutely phenomenal at what they do. Their knowledge of diseases and pathological processes is amazing. The staggering number of drugs, both generic and name brand that they prescribe is unbelievable in its complexity. The number and kinds of tests and procedures that they must have knowledge of and be able to rattle off at any given moment is phenomenal. But the definition of wellness is an absence of disease. Just because a person isn't currently ill with a specific disease or pathological condition, doesn't mean that they are healthy and in the best physical condition that they can be. A person trying to attain true wellness may not find the best advice coming from their overworked physician.

Wellness means trying to be as healthy as one can be, not just for the sake of not being ill, but for the sake of wellness itself. The healthier one is, the healthier one should remain and the faster one should recover if illness should unfortunately strike them. Most physicians today are kept so busy treating pathology and genuinely sick people that they have little time to concern themselves with wellness, or helping you to achieve excellent health.

The hairstylist with bad hair has the same license hanging on her wall as the hairstylist who does an excellent, careful and detailed job. The paint company that has a dirty beat up work truck with ragged lettering in the windows can likely do the same job as the one with a clean, well maintained truck with crisp lettering. The person you choose to paint your house or cut and style your hair is up to you. It is entirely up to you, as a consumer, to make the choice as to which hairstylist or painter will do a better job on your hair or on your house. The same goes for dietary and exercise advice.

If you want to improve your health and be skinny and fit, you need advice from someone who lives that lifestyle and is thin and healthy themselves. If this does not describe your physician, you likely need to get your dietary and exercise advice from someone else.

You should continue to get your medical advice from your physician. A good knowledgeable physician, of any weight and health, is hard to find, and if you currently have an excellent physician, by all means maintain that connection. But consider getting your exercise and nutrition information elsewhere. It will always be prudent to run by any drastic changes with someone who is medically trained, knows you well and that you trust, but I don't know many physicians today who have a whole lot of time to sit down and discuss matters of maintaining excellent health and wellness with their patient's.

Physicians today are rewarded by and expected to treat pathology and disease. There is very little pay or incentive for them to work to keep you from becoming ill in the first place. If the standard set of tests that they run shows that all of your results are within the "normal" range, they will be finished with your care until the next year. You may not be truly "well" but if your numbers are in the normal range or close to it, they will quickly move on to someone who needs their services much more, the sick and the unwell. There are plenty of ill people in the United States to keep all of our physicians working long hours. Keeping you from becoming ill or truly being well is supposed to be the focus of medical practice but often there are so many people with more serious pathology that will require their advanced care that they will be happy to place a check mark next to your name, and move right along.

When I was majoring in biology during my undergraduate studies at Christopher Newport University in Newport News, Virginia, I took a class called Human Nutrition. As the professor introduced the course he told us that after we had finished the class we would know more about nutrition than the average physician does. He told us that the role of medical schools is to train physicians to recognize disease processes. From there they are to make a proper diagnosis and begin a treatment with either a drug regimen or surgical intervention. All of this is to improve the pathology the patient is suffering from. Medical school only lasts four years with the last two years spent in clinical rotations. That leaves two years for a physician to learn everything there is to know about the human body, recognize all known pathological states, and memorize all of the drug treatments and what they do and how they should be prescribed. That is a lot of information. There simply isn't time for a physician's schedule to contain extra nutrition and exercise courses.

When I asked my physician if my flaking skin condition could be related to my diet, he told me that it was highly unlikely and even if it was he didn't think the average person would actually stop eating foods that are likely harmful, even if they knew what those foods were. He said that people are usually unwilling to implement a strategy of dietary control as part of a legitimate treatment plan. Besides, he said, it was easier to use the drugs than try to change someone's dietary habits which are deeply ingrained and unlikely to change for the long term. I would have been happy to take his advice and leave it at that if the prescribed medical treatments would have worked. But unfortunately, the drugs only relieved my symptoms by thirty percent or so. After carefully following his advice, I was still pretty miserable and I thought that there had to be a better way.

Another disturbing trend that I discovered while undertaking this dietary change concerns the often bothersome physical traits known as menopause. All women in the United States are expected to undergo a drastic change to their bodies between the ages of forty and sixty as their ovaries markedly slow down their production of the hormone estrogen. This is usually a period of time in which a woman undergoes significant changes to her body. Most of these changes are not good except for the fact that she can no longer become pregnant. This period of time is supposed to be filled with anxiety, night sweats, unexpected weight gain, breast tenderness and general feelings of inadequacy and questioning of self-worth.

A quick trip to the doctor's office with a description of these symptoms in hand will cause the physician to give you a prescription for Premarin, which is a drug made from the urine of pregnant horses. This drug increases the hormone estrogen in the body to counteract the effects of the ovaries decreasing their release of estrogen. This drug replaces the estrogen that the ovaries were producing with the estrogen produced by a pregnant horse and causes a rise in the estrogen level in the body to counteract the decrease in estrogen. Eating the rich western diet, full of meat, eggs and dairy products that all include estrogen, causes the bodies of women and girls who eat these products to have much more estrogen in their bodies than women in countries where consumption of these products is not as common. In menopause, the sharp drop in estrogen levels available in the body leads to the night sweats, fatigue and malaise. In countries where the excess estrogen is not present, the women still experience a drop in estrogen levels but it is not so drastic that they become symptomatic.

If you are still fairly young, the doctor will give you birth-control pills and tell you that it's okay to take them for several more years, even though the warning label on them states that if you take them over the age of thirty-five your risk for heart attacks and strokes markedly increases when taking these drugs. An even newer trend is to give women who complain of menopausal symptoms psychiatric drugs, like anti-depressants. Seriously, who wouldn't be depressed with these kinds of symptoms and doesn't this just reinforce the old stereotypical thinking that all women are crazy, anyway?

What I found interesting in my research is that in countries where the consumption of meat, dairy products, caffeine and processed sugar are low, they do not actually have a word for menopause. What? How can this be? Why would they not have a word to describe menopause? After undergoing a serious diet change myself and eating only healthy foods for a very long period of time I now know why they don't have a word to describe menopause. It is because the symptoms of menopause are magnified with a diet high in meat, dairy, eggs, processed white sugar, white flour, caffeine and junk food.

That's right. Can you believe that? How come the doctor doesn't just tell us if we stop eating a bunch of garbage our body will feel much better? How come eating a rich and junk food filled diet leads to increased symptoms of menopause? I have enough scientific knowledge to know that this is true but I cannot describe the phenomenon that actually takes place within the body regarding this.. After researching it for some time it seems that nobody else can either. The research seems to indicate that the drop in estrogen triggers an area of the brain where the thermostat of the body is kept, causing the hot flashing sensation as the body works to regulate the temperature. Nobody knows why this occurs. That's right. We can put a man on the moon but cannot understand why the thermoregulation system in women gets all messed up when they go through menopause...hmm...

Women who live in countries where mostly plant foods and unprocessed grains are consumed do not even experience enough menopause symptoms to give the feeling a word. They have no description for this phenomenon. It can't be because they don't have anything to say. It has to be because they are not experiencing the same symptoms. Why are they not experiencing these symptoms? Could it be that between the ages of forty and sixty our bodies are simply responding to a heightened state of hormonal activity? All of the research in this area seems to indicate that the least amount of hormone that the body is exposed to during this time of life the better the outcome is for us as far as heart disease and all other causes of mortality is.

It used to be that every single physician would simply give women a prescription for estrogen, thinking that they were helping them, until research was done in this area which proved quite the opposite. In fact the research in this area was so compelling that the study was actually stopped before it was completed. Physicians are now in a bind when it comes to this sort of thing as women presenting to their office expect something to be done about these miserable hot flashes, breast tenderness, anxiety and night sweats.

A woman undergoing this kind of event naturally feels extremely sorry for herself as her body undergoes these changes. Wouldn't it be amazing if this was all caused by an improper diet? Can you imagine what a relief it is to find that this is not the normal state of being for a woman between the ages of forty and sixty? By eating properly and exercising regularly, a woman can avoid most of these symptoms. I'm sure you have witnessed women undergoing this drastic life change and you have seen how they break out and sweat for no reason and experience skin breakouts and anxiety as a result of these hormonal upheavals. They appear extremely uncomfortable and this is a very socially awkward phenomena. Wouldn't it be amazing if this could all be avoided by eating and exercising properly? It just seems ridiculously easy. Further research needs to be done in this field but it would certainly be wonderful to find that menopause symptoms, which seem to go on and on and on for several years in some susceptible individuals, can be laid permanently to rest with a few months of a good diet and three to five hours a week of exercise.

On the opposite side of this spectrum are the hormonal changes that take place in adolescents. Puberty used to be a phenomenon that occurred after thirteen to fifteen years of age in males and females. The age at which puberty occurs has been steadily going down for a number of years. Our country right now is in a state where little girls are beginning to menstruate as early as eight years old on a regular basis. What could be causing this? I have heard that it could possibly be the fluorescent lights, the GMO's, overconsumption of fast food junk, etc.

Again, there is no scientific data to back this up, but my belief is that this, too, is caused by an over exposure to the added hormones in the meat, dairy and eggs. The cows that provide nearly all of the milk supplied in this country are kept pregnant and lactating at the same time, a phenomenon that did not used to be the case. With children being told and encouraged to drink milk four times a day and with the increase in cheese and ice cream consumption, there is no question in my mind that this "over nutrition" with an emphasis on excessive protein, is also causing this epidemic of unnaturally early puberty.

Breast feeding children exclusively for the first six months to one year of life is talked about and encouraged, but unfortunately, not necessarily done. This causes even infants to be exposed to cows' milk protein from the very beginning, setting them up for early puberty, obesity and illness.

There is also a concern that exposing susceptible children to dairy products before the age of two could be responsible for the onset of Type 1 diabetes, as the milk protein leaks through the immature gut wall of a young child, causing an immune system reaction.

The cells on the pancreas, where the insulin is created, are called Beta cells. These Beta cells look an awful lot like cow's milk protein. The theory is that the body's immune system is triggered when the cow's milk protein comes through the naturally "leaky gut" of a young child. From there, the body's immune system continues to fight this cow's milk protein and then attacks the insulin secreting Beta cells of the pancreas as well in an unfortunate "friendly fire" type incident. The Beta cells are then destroyed and a child develops Type 1, or what used to be called Juvenile onset, diabetes.

A child's gut or intestinal wall is naturally "leaky" to allow the antibodies present in the child's mothers milk to stimulate the child's immune system naturally. This "leaky gut" lasts for the first two years or so of a child's life.

Feeding children properly would go a long way towards preserving their childhood and preventing serious illnesses. The longer it takes for a girl to begin menstruating, the taller she will be, and the less her body will be exposed to too much estrogen, which should decrease the incidence in our population of hormone responsive cancers and decrease the severity of puberty and menopause symptoms when this child is an adult as well.

Eating properly is important for our entire lifespans. So many people would be helped if children were simply fed properly and never given cow's milk at least until the age of two. So many cases of Type 1 diabetes could be prevented by simply breast feeding infants properly. So much heartache and tragedy could be prevented. Can you imagine a world without diabetes, type 1 or type 2, without acne, obesity and without menopausal symptoms? This is all very likely possible with proper nutrition.

As part of the nutrition class that I was enrolled in, each of the students was given a computer program and was asked to track their food intake over a week or so and use the database to see how it compared to the USDA (United States Department of Agriculture) recommendations and guidelines.

What I learned from keeping track of the foods that I ate and analyzing the nutritional content in my nutrition class was that most of the food I ate had almost no nutritional value whatsoever. Every day when I entered the foods that I had eaten, believing it to be a normal and healthful diet, I never met the daily requirements for more than one or two nutrients. Not even one day out of the whole week. And my intake of fat, saturated fat, and cholesterol were all way over where they were supposed to be, and I was a vegetarian.

I recognized it as a problem at the time but didn't really know what to do about it. The answer seemed to be just to not eat anything at all and take vitamin supplements, which of course is ridiculous. I remember wondering at the time what could be done about it and thinking to myself that it was strange. Even then it did not occur to me to simply add fruits, vegetables and whole grains to my diet. I think this was because the USDA guidelines were talking about components of food instead of listing the actual names of appropriate foods to eat.

Like many people that I know, I had read several newspaper and magazine articles, as well as learning in the nutrition class, that if I ate a generally balanced "normal" American diet I had nothing to fear as far as nutritional deprivation as over the course of a few days I likely took in all of the nutrients my body required and then some. We have all been reassured over and over that the United States doesn't have a malnutrition problem and thankfully hasn't had one for years and years. As long as I kept my intake of all foods "in moderation" I had nothing to fear.

The nutrition class I was taking focused on the food pyramid that was being promoted by the USDA at the time. At the time it was thought that one should eat six to eleven servings of grains, two to three servings of vegetables and fruits, two to three servings of meat, three to four servings of dairy and use fats, sweets and oils sparingly. I never ate all of the required foods or even came close to meeting any of the requirements. I did however take note that if I actually ate the amount of food recommended by the government I would easily weigh three hundred pounds. I mean three cups of milk (one hundred fifty calories each), six to eleven servings of bread and grain (one hundred fifty calories each) and two to three servings of meat (one hundred fifty to three hundred calories each) would easily pack one thousand six hundred or more calories with the lowest available serving sizes and that was before I added fruit and vegetables and of course all of the usual tasty favorite treats I ate on a regular basis to get me through the day and fill me with energy, such as soda and potato chips.

While looking at these recommendations, all of a sudden, a nation struggling with obesity makes sense. At this time the USDA has changed their standards somewhat and is currently using a thing called "My Plate" which is completely confusing to even a trained person.

In the back of most American's heads is the fact that one MUST eat from the various food groups (Milk, Meat, Grains, Vegetables and Fruits) or possibly suffer serious malnutrition as a result. Especially ingrained in the American mindset is the idea that getting enough protein is paramount to good health. Since meat, milk, yogurt, eggs and cheese contain protein, they form the backbone of a standard American diet. This was taught to most Americans receiving a public education somewhere in the elementary grades and emphasized several times in health courses through the rest of school. "You have to get enough protein" as enough protein is paramount to good health, or at least this is the thought process I remember learning about.

So after I had taken this college level nutrition class, I did what most Americans do and I ignored the pyramid, I ignored My Plate and I just ate what was easy and tasted good, occasionally swallowing a few multivitamins thinking that is what I was supposed to do to make myself feel better. Taking the multivitamins did not physically make me feel better.

But I was worried about all of the conflicting information. Information on nutrition is usually thrown at us in the headlines and then we are often left not sure what to do. "Multivitamins cause cancer" screamed the headlines. "Eat more fish." "Fish are tainted with mercury" "Vitamin D Deficiency and Osteoporosis are rampant in the United States". "Drink more coffee", "cholesterol levels don't matter", etc.

To cope with the stress in my life as a working mom and student with two young sons, and to keep me alert enough to perform my job, I usually drank three or more cola beverages every day. The caffeine gave me energy and the sugar made me feel better. When I started going to physical therapy school, my fellow students pointed out how terrible it was to drink full sugar soda and as a result I thought I would be healthy and switched to diet cola. After all these drinks didn't have any calories, how bad could they be? They are FDA approved.

Everything I read about it seemed to indicate that this was not a problem, so I kept it up. Easily available research didn't indicate any issues with consuming soda daily or even several times per day, for that matter, especially diet soda. I had constant stomach pain and sometimes in the middle of the night, my stomach would hurt enough that I couldn't go back to sleep for several hours until I got up and swallowed some over the counter pain relievers. I thought I just had irritable bowel syndrome that wasn't really serious enough to warrant seeing a physician. My skin had patches of eczema that I would treat with lotions and by eating more fish with occasional trips to the dermatologist for more prescriptions. As a physical therapist I worked through my constant fatigue and exercised three days a week to maintain my reputation as a fitness expert.

The breaking point health wise and weight wise happened to me when I needed to undergo an elective outpatient surgery. At the time of my surgery, I had been dieting at 1200 – 1400 calories a day diet for several weeks and running on my treadmill for two to five miles per day, three to five days a week, usually between fifteen and twenty miles per week. I weighed around 140 pounds and at 5'4" tall my BMI was 24.0. At my pre-op checkup my blood pressure was high enough (160 / 90) that my surgeon was concerned.

I know that I have a tendency to over react to many things. I know that I am what is typically known as a "hot reactor". This means that when I am in a situation that I find stressful, instead of being mildly stressed, I completely spaz out! This was the likely cause of the increased blood pressure reading. I tried to explain to the physician that it was just fear and a weird physical reaction to the increased psychological stress of the upcoming surgery but my physician was really worried about it. The physician who was treating me had me lie in a dark room with my feet elevated for twenty minutes and came back to obtain a second blood pressure reading which had actually raised from 160/ 90 to 180 / 95. As a result of this reading he placed me on medication to lower my blood pressure and advised me to follow up with a cardiologist after my upcoming surgery for further treatment of my hypertension.

After two days of taking the prescribed medicine I was so ill I could hardly work. My heart was beating rapidly at 120 beats per minute, (up from its usual 90) and I felt dizzy and ill and as a result my anxiety was even worse. I stopped taking the medication, my heart rate returned to 90 and I immediately felt better but continued to suffer from anxiety induced hypertension.

The day before my surgery I ran five miles on a treadmill to try and get my blood pressure low enough so that I would be able to undergo the surgical procedure the next day. On the day of the surgery my blood pressure was sky high and I explained to the surgical prep team what I thought was going on and I heard them whispering in the hall way about how they remembered me from a previous medical procedure and that my blood pressure would stabilize as soon as I was given the amnesiac medication and of course, it did. My blood pressure came down to 130 / 80 and my heart rate to 85. These are "normal" numbers but definitely not healthy numbers.

At my follow up visit following the surgery, my doctor suggested that my problem was likely "white coat syndrome" in which a person's blood pressure climbs as a result of just thinking about undergoing a medical procedure. He then showed me an article in a medical journal which stated that white coat syndrome was actually a precursor to real hypertension. It certainly would make sense that I might be coming down with real hypertension.

My parents both have hypertension as did my grandmother. Although my weight was around one hundred forty pounds this was the upper limit of normal for a person of my height. Hypertension seemed a likely legitimate diagnosis based on the evidence. My heart was fluttery and I noticed an occasional sensation like it had skipped a beat. Despite the fact that I regularly did cardiovascular exercise, my resting heart rate was still quite high, usually between 85-90 beats per minute. My weight varied between one hundred forty and one hundred forty three pounds which I carried well. People told me that I looked good. But the truth was that my pants and clothing were getting too tight in the waist. My size ten pants were turning into size twelve's. I did not look good in a swimsuit.

This was very discouraging as I had an entire wardrobe of size ten clothing that I really enjoyed wearing. I kind of rationalized it in my mind saying that on a scale from one to ten I was a ten and therefore I wore a size ten. This analogy didn't make any sense for a size twelve. So I decided to declare major war on my body in an attempt to get my weight and body to comply back in the size ten that I was used to wearing.

As I recovered from my surgery I put myself on a stricter diet, limiting myself to no more than 1200 calories a day of any kind of food that I wanted. After all I had been told over and over again that a calorie is a calorie whatever the source, and I believed it. 3500 calories in a pound of fat.

Burn it off or don't eat it and there you go, a pound gone. At least that was my mindset at the time.

I also became even more regimented about my treadmill running and ran religiously three to four days per week, covering five miles per session. After six weeks of this I had not lost a single pound. After three months of this I had lost five pounds. I went from a weight of one hundred forty three pounds to one hundred thirty eight pounds. I had lost only five pounds!

As I previously discussed, I felt deprived, very hungry and cold most of the time. I did my best to not be irritable but I was very cranky from depriving myself of everything. The only thing I had to look forward on a daily basis was my two hundred calorie cup of 7-Eleven French Vanilla Cappuccino and a small serving of either white pasta and marinara sauce with canned green beans or a small amount of corn chips and salsa that I ate almost nightly. I thought canned vegetables were equally as nutritious as any other kind. They were convenient and easy. The people selling canned vegetables had even advertised this as being true.

About this time I was also feeling like my eyes just wouldn't stay open and they were so dry I felt like I needed constant eye drops just to get through the day. I was experiencing episodes where my skin felt so dry and itchy and my throat hurt all day every day. I had sinus congestion that I thought must be allergy induced.

After a few months of this misery I went to a physician who was an ear nose throat specialist and he advised allergy testing which I did. The stunning and spectacular results of this testing showed that I was allergic to absolutely nothing! How could this be? Why was my nose running constantly? Why did I catch every cold on the planet? Why was I freezing cold all of the time? Why were my skin and eyes so itchy and dry that I could barely stand getting through each day? This all made me very frustrated.

I do have Hashimoto's thyroiditis but I took my daily thyroid medication as my endocrinologist physician advised. That problem was being addressed so the symptoms should have been gone. At one hundred thirty eight pounds and after three months of very serious calorie restriction and exercise I stopped my diet.

I resumed my normal eating patterns and almost immediately I regained the five hard fought pounds. The hypertension scare was really bothering me as was my chronically elevated heart rate. The weird blood pressure elevation, the eczema, the heart pounding out of my chest when I wasn't even exercising, weren't these signs of some kind of illness? I felt like there had to be something wrong. I wasn't happy about these problems but there didn't seem to be anything I could do about this. I knew I could not stand another restricted calorie diet and with my busy schedule I was running for exercise as much as I could. Exercise should have made me skinny and it wasn't working. This couldn't be normal. This just didn't make any sense.

At the same time all of this was happening to me, my husband was fighting a similar battle. Having been diagnosed with thyroid cancer at the age of thirty nine, he had his thyroid gland removed and was also taking thyroid medication.

In his youth he had been a trim one hundred fifty to one hundred sixty five pounds but after leaving the army and being self- employed, his weight had continued to rise and at 5'11" tall his weight had risen to two hundred forty five pounds. He was in the process of trading up his size thirty eight waist pants for a forty inch waist. He had been diagnosed with Type II diabetes six years earlier and his doctor was also concerned about hypertension and high cholesterol. He was told that he would soon begin medication to manage these diseases as well.

At the time he was also taking an unusually large dose of Allopurinol to manage his chronic gout symptoms, which he had been battling since his late twenties. The results of his A1C test, the test that physicians' use to see how well a person has been able to control their blood sugar fluctuations in the past three months, was 8.9 and this was not good, even with him taking the medication Metformin for his diabetes twice a day.

I knew that he was taking the medication as prescribed because it was my job to make sure that he took his medication as he would just "forget" every day if I didn't follow him around with the pills and a glass of water. He had to take a Synthroid, for his thyroid, when he woke up in the morning, a Metformin, for diabetes, right after lunch and then another Metformin right after supper and then an Allopurinol, for his gout, before bed.

Things had gotten so out of control that his physician told him that if he didn't get his A1C test under control, to 7 or less, that they would have to start considering the use of daily insulin to control his excess blood sugar and the doctor wanted him to take a cholesterol lowering medication and a medication for hypertension as well.

This all sounded like a complete nightmare to me. I was having enough difficulty getting him to take his thyroid medicine, his diabetes medicine and his gout medicine and trying to get him to actually test his blood sugar was impossible. Sometimes I would hand him a pill and have his glass of water ready and he would take them from me and I would come back a few hours later to see the pill lying on the counter with the glass of water next to it. He was like a prison inmate. I had to actually physically watch him take the pills or it wouldn't happen! Here was this man that I loved and cared for deeply suffering from all of these illnesses and he wasn't even fifty years old. I knew that there was no way I could go on like this, with me acting as the prison warden actually watching him swallow his pills several times a day.

All of a sudden something inside of me snapped. I couldn't take it anymore. We were in our very early forties and looking at years of medications and side effects and I just couldn't believe this could be happening to us. I resolved to find out how to solve my problems and his problems. My quest led me to the plan you will find outlined in this book. I loved my husband way too much to watch him become sick and old from all of these chronic conditions and diseases. I loved myself way too much to become another chubby mother carting her kids around from activity to activity.

I couldn't take it anymore! This was insanity! It is said that the definition of insanity is doing the same thing over and over and expecting a different result. Obviously counting calories and running constantly were not working. I was ready to do something different. I was finished with insanity.

Now I want to admit right here that I am a vegetarian. I have been a vegetarian for many, many years. People become vegetarians for different reasons and my reason is that I have always felt a great deal of compassion for all living creatures. Just like Dr. Doolittle in the old fashioned movie starring Rex Harrison, I just simply cannot eat my very best friends. My vegetarianism was not for health reasons. I simply feel, and continue to feel very strongly, that I cannot and should not eat animals for ethical reasons of my own.

With that being said, I am not judgmental of others who eat meat on a regular basis and although I am slightly grossed out when others are eating meat in my presence, I work very hard not to be judgmental about it. I actually admire people who hunt and fish and then eat what they catch and kill as they are the only meat eaters who truly know what happened to their meat before they ate it. At least they are honest about what they are doing. Do I think that they need to kill animals to provide themselves with food? Of course they do not. And of course I do not believe they are providing themselves or their families with anything even close to ideal nutrition. Hunting and fishing are cultural practices for many people. I know very few other vegetarians in my immediate circle of friends and acquaintances and am always surprised and pleased to meet others who share my views.

People can be so very cruel to animals. I have always deeply loved animals and have always been very mindful of their existence and to the fact that there used to be a body with a personality attached to the steak, chicken, fish and shrimp on my plate. I have been exposed to chickens and a goose being slaughtered in my childhood which had affected me deeply. I find killing and eating animals deeply disturbing and felt the same horror about these events as I did when the neighbors announced that they had thrown a litter of kittens into the river tied in a plastic bag as they could not care for any more animals. I feel that there is absolutely no difference between the animals that are frequently eaten by human beings and the ones that are frequently kept as pets. They are all precious and I could never bring myself to eat their dead bodies.

When I decided to become a vegetarian, at the age of twenty seven, this was a big shock to my family and especially to my mother who truly thought that I might actually die from a lack of protein in my diet. I continued to eat fish and shrimp once or twice a week to appease her and to try and stop the constant dry itching skin that was on my legs, which I thought, could possibly be caused by a lack of protein. I was horrified to think that she might be right (as mothers often are). It wasn't until later that I discovered I was technically a pescatarian, or one who eats fish and seafood, but no land animals. I ate the fish and seafood as I felt they were essential to my health but I was not happy about it. From that day until now I have never eaten any beef, pork or chicken.

After beginning my new plan and in the process of researching this book and as a result of my now very healthy vegan diet, I chose to never again eat seafood. I am so relieved that it is not a necessary part of my diet or anyone else's for that matter. Most people that I know and regularly associate with continue to eat meat and animal

7

containing foods on a regular basis to this day. This book is not about vegetarianism. You do not need to be a vegetarian to eat healthfully. It will certainly help to limit meat and all animal containing foods to very small (one to two ounce) portions no more than one to two days per month, but you do not have to give it up entirely. My vegetarianism is a philosophical point of view that I do for ethical reasons of my own.

With that being said, it is sometimes easier to give something up entirely than to eat it in very small quantities that become very large quantities when you cannot think of anything else to eat. I guess this would be like a smoker who smokes one to two cigarettes a month. It is possible to do so and hardly suffer from the health problems that cigarettes cause but very difficult to actually be a one to two cigarette a month smoker due to the highly addictive nature of nicotine. A similar problem exists for people who eat animal products on a regular basis.

If you have been a meat eater on a regular basis and are used to eating meat or animal containing foods with nearly every meal, it may be easier to just not eat it at all, at least for the first six weeks, so that you can train yourself to look for other options. You are going to have to be the judge of your own feelings on this subject. If you can tolerate eating very small, and I do mean, very small servings of meat or other animal products and only eating them rarely, only once or twice per month at most, then you should feel free to continue this practice once or twice a month as long as your health parameters (blood pressure, cholesterol, weight, heart rate, blood sugar, etc.) are all normal. You cannot eat animal products all day, every day, several times per day and be healthy. It just isn't possible.

My permission for you to eat animal containing foods is only for those individuals who feel emotionally comfortable killing and or paying someone else to kill living creatures on their behalf. You also must already have a BMI of between 18.5 – 23.0 if you are a woman and between 20 and 25.0 if you are a man, maintain a cholesterol level under 150 without medications, have a resting heart rate of less than 65 beats per minute, have fasting blood sugar tests of under 100 and have blood pressure readings of 110 / 70 or lower. When these goals are met without the use of any medications to maintain them, a person can eat meat and animal products "in moderation", meaning once or twice a month if they do not have a philosophical problem with eating other sentient beings.

Everyone else should abstain from eating animals or animal containing products until these parameters are also met for them. These measurements are goals that need to be met in order to attain true wellness.

Because of their high calorie content and their poor nutritional makeup, meat and animal containing foods are poor food choices. They are calorically dense and contain an exceptional amount of fat, especially saturated fat, and cholesterol and have minimal nutritional value. They are just not a nutrient dense form of calories. This eating plan is all about obtaining enough nutrients to make your body truly well and healthy. If you feel that you have to eat a large portion of meat, several times a day, several days a week, you will never be thin and even if you manage to be thin you will never be healthy. There may be one to two percent of the population that is able to maintain the healthy biological measurements listed above while eating anything that they want, but for the majority of us, it just is not possible.

I have met very few people, perhaps one or two, over the age of thirty five that are skinny and fit and continue to eat meat and other animal containing products on a regular basis. I have seen most people become thin for short periods of time, then regain their lost weight, sometimes repeatedly, but I have never seen them start overweight and lose weight, obtaining and maintaining a good and healthy weight with normal blood pressure, cholesterol level under 150, heart rate under 65, blood pressure under 110/70 and normal A1C's for years on end while eating animal containing food on a regular basis. I have seen some that are naturally thin, but their biological measurements are pathological. I have seen some of them become thinner but then still have health problems and have to take medication to control hypertension and high cholesterol. I have seen them become thinner but still have stubborn belly fat that sticks around. Eating meat and animal containing foods on a regular basis is just a way that is guaranteed to make you fat and sick.

If you have to eat animal containing foods all of the time, every day, then this plan just will not work for you. Please understand that human nutrition does not require the consumption of animal products and nothing bad will happen to you if you give them up entirely. So many people are deathly afraid that they will die or become ill if they don't constantly eat animals and / or animal products. I promise nothing bad will happen to you. In fact you will actually recover from many chronic illnesses and lose weight in a healthy way. This is a guarantee. The only nutrient you need concern yourself with is Vitamin B12, which everyone, meat eater or not, should take anyway.

With my initial change to a vegetarian (but not vegan) diet, I didn't really notice much of a change in my health or weight although when I had routine cholesterol screening my cholesterol was 230. I, like many people in this country, have a family history of elevated cholesterol. When I say high, I mean HIGH. For instance my mother has a cholesterol level of 385 without medication. My grandmother's was 450. This is really high. In this country a normal cholesterol reading is considered to be at or below 200 although research into this number led me to realize that this is just an arbitrary number that doesn't really mean anything. Scientific research has shown that a truly healthy cholesterol reading is a cholesterol level below 150, which is really needed to prevent heart disease.

In my case, my physician wasn't concerned about my high cholesterol because at the time my HDL (high density lipoprotein) level was 110. HDL is considered to be "good" cholesterol. This was likely as a result of my vegetarian diet or the running that I do or maybe a combination of the two. My identical twin sister's cholesterol was 270 at the same time. Now when I say I switched to a vegetarian diet at the age of twenty seven, that doesn't mean I ate lots of fruit, vegetables and beans. Mostly I continued to eat the things I always had, just without the meat. This included lots of white pasta, white bread and crackers and tomato sauce, cheese pizza, yogurt, and tons of easily accessible processed food just like most American's eat on a daily basis.

The diet I currently eat is vegan, with whole foods as much as possible and without added oil. I do not ever eat the flesh of any animal, as a matter of personal principle and I strongly feel that is just not possible to become thin and maintain a thin physique eating animal products or meat on a regular basis, especially if you are over thirty five years old. It is much easier to become slim and remain slim when meat eating is kept to a very small minimum, meaning one two small (one to two ounce) servings per month.

Again, I personally do not eat ANY animals, not fish, not chicken, not seafood of any kind and my one to two servings a month or less of animal product related foods are limited to the whipped topping on top of a dessert or beverage or the eggs mixed into pancake batter, cookies, bread or pasta, all eaten at a restaurant or outside of my home. I do not consume any animals or animal containing foods in my home. I do not cook with them or use them at all. I don't cook with animal products at home and I don't eat or use animal products or added oils or fats at all while I am cooking at home.

I just want it to be very clear that animal containing foods offer protein, yes, but without any other real benefit. Animal based foods do not contain any other type of known vitamin or nutrient that is required by the human body that cannot better be obtained in plant based foods with the exception of Vitamin B12. Animal products contain an awful lot of calories and fat for the protein that they provide and they tend to contain many substances that raise cholesterol and in general cause or exacerbate chronic health problems, like inflammation.

There are many, many better alternatives and options for obtaining protein in the human diet than by eating animals or animal containing foods. All of the alternatives are much better suited to our nutritional needs as humans and do not come in packages that also contain dangerous substances. So the real question is why do people eat so many animal products? I think the majority of American's eat animal containing foods all day every day simply out of habit.

For the purposes of this plan, animal products will be considered junk food. This is because of their inferior nutritional profile. For the purpose of this plan animal products or animal containing foods are not going to be considered as part of a healthy diet but instead will be seen as part of the "flavoring" agents or very occasional treats that some people need in order to live happy and fulfilled lives. Again, let me emphasize that I am not one of those people and would gladly do without them completely but I do understand that that is not a majority opinion in our country at this time and having people markedly reduce their consumption of these types of foods will significantly affect their health in a positive way and is much better than getting caught up in a dogmatic all or nothing approach that doesn't solve any one's health problems and leaves people feeling angry, left out and frustrated. I believe that there is room for all of us to work together to improve the health of this nation.

Every time someone finds out that I do not eat any animal products the first question they ask me is where do I get my protein. I get my protein from the same place that all of the other animals get their protein, like the very large cows, the elephants and the giraffes. I get my protein from plants. Obviously there is a lot of protein in beans, but did you know that most green vegetables are pretty close to fifty percent protein as well? "What?..." I can almost hear you saying. "How can this be?"

I will bet that most people are completely unaware of this fact. Yes. This is the truth. Green vegetables, including broccoli, romaine lettuce, spinach and kale are close to fifty percent protein. Not only do they contain protein but they also contain a very high amount of other vitamins, phytochemicals and micronutrients, not to mention fiber, which we humans need in order for our bodies to function normally.

Isn't this shocking? Isn't this amazing? Why isn't this common knowledge? I was surprised myself. So after years of being a vegetarian, after discovering this truth, I actually began to really eat vegetables and fruit.

I now believe that vegetables, especially the green ones, should make up part of our daily diet. I get my protein, and plenty of it, in fact all that I need and then some more, from the green vegetables and other plant products like grains and beans that are in my diet, just like the giraffe, the cow, the horse and you should too.

If, after eating without animal products, you feel that something is missing from your diet, the solution is to eat MORE of this very nutritious and healthy food. Eat until you are full, not stuffed, but satisfied.

The next question people ask me when they find out that I do not eat any animal products is what about calcium? Won't you get osteoporosis if you don't drink your milk or eat dairy products? Most people think that you simply must have milk in order to grow strong, healthy bones.

Nope. That turns out to not be true either. Most green vegetables and many different fruits, beans and sesame seeds have quite a lot of calcium in them too! That is where the very large land mammals, such as elephants and giraffes, not to mention cows, get their calcium to grow their very large bones from. They get it from the green things that grow in the ground! I have never run into a large land mammal suffering from osteoporosis except for human beings! In fact, only humans who live an affluent lifestyle with plenty of meat and plenty of milk ever seem to get osteoporosis.

An African village woman who eats a very near vegan diet can give birth to eight children, breast feed all of them for years and still have all of her teeth and good posture at the age of sixty. How could this be possible as she never drinks milk? It is because of the green vegetables that she eats. Remember, we are just big, fancy primates and what do primates eat? They eat vegetables and fruits and lots and lots of them.

Do you know what really causes osteoporosis? Osteoporosis is likely caused by acidic blood pH. The pH scale runs from 0 – 14 with 7 indicating a neutral pH. Plain water is supposed to be 7.0 on the pH scale. Anything that is under a pH of 7 is called acidic. Anything over a pH of 7 is called basic or alkaline. The blood in the body is meant to be maintained at a pH level of 7.45, which is slightly basic, or alkaline, at all times. If our blood chemistry is not maintained at this 7.45 pH level, very serious pathology, illness and death will soon result.

A known problem with a diet which is made up of meat, milk, cheese, yogurt and eggs is that it decreases the pH level of the blood, which then becomes slightly acidic. The body knows that this cannot be tolerated and uses calcium as a buffering agent to buffer the blood and maintain a constant pH level of 7.45, which is slightly alkaline. Anyone who has taken a basic chemistry class or has an aquarium or pool knows that calcium is an excellent buffering agent used to adjust pH upwards.

Guess where the body gets the calcium needed to buffer the acidic blood? Guess where there is a great big store of calcium that the body can easily access? That's right, in your bones. This is high school chemistry. So osteoporosis appears to be caused by an excessive intake of protein from animal derived foods that cause the pH of the blood to trend downwards towards being acidic, so the body has to use calcium in the bones to buffer the acidic blood and return it to its normally slightly basic or alkaline state of

7.45 on the pH scale. This, combined with a lack of weight bearing exercise, contributes strongly to osteoporosis.

Our bodies operate on a "use or lose it" principle. If you never do any weight bearing exercise, then your body feels that it is unnecessary to keep a heavy skeleton when a light one will work. A lack of weight bearing exercise combined with a mostly acidic food intake is what is causing this huge osteoporosis epidemic. (Br J Nutr. 2010 Apr; 103(8):1185-94. doi: 10.1017/S0007114509993047. Epub 2009 Dec 15.Diet-induced acidosis: is it real and clinically relevant?Pizzorno J1, Frassetto LA, Katzinger J.)

Doesn't this sound like the typical American diet and lifestyle? I think it sounds exactly like the way we live. We are living a lifestyle that promotes osteoporosis and then wondering how this could be happening. Osteoporosis is at its worst in countries that consume the highest levels of meat and milk and is almost nonexistent where the people do not eat this kind of diet.

The consumption of meat, milk and eggs appears to CAUSE osteoporosis and not prevent it. Milk doesn't make it better, it makes it worse. Research has shown that a diet that contains more than sixteen percent of its calories from animal based protein causes the blood pH to decrease, or become acidic, and causes calcium to be excreted in the urine even faster than it can be brought in. Even if a person were to drink two or more quarts of milk a day, the calcium lost in the person's urine would still be greater than the amount being taken in by the drinking of the milk, with the result being a net loss of calcium. If this trend were to continue, it would eventually lead to osteoporosis. In eating an abundance of rich, protein containing foods that are derived from animal products we are literally "peeing" our bones right out of our bodies and wondering why we have kidney stones while we do it.

So, to summarize, your physician is very good at his or her job, which is understanding and recognizing disease and disease processes, diagnosing and treating them accurately and quickly and referring you to a specialist when a specialist is needed.

Unless your physician is pretty unusual, he or she is not usually as good at keeping people healthy or working with them to restore their health with diet and exercise. He or she is already overworked and doing the best that he or she can do to properly care for the truly sick people in his or her care. There is no financial incentive for your physician to keep you healthy. He or she will not get paid to teach you how to eat properly or when prescribing a diet of carrots and apples. It is not that your physician doesn't care, he or she cares very deeply, he simply doesn't have the time, energy and often does not have the knowledge to devote to these concepts when there are so many, very sick people that need to be treated and cared for.

Choose your physician carefully, and never be afraid to consult with him or her if you are concerned about health matters, but don't expect your physician to know how the average person can obtain excellent health. Physicians simply don't have the time to spend making you well. Don't be afraid to discuss the contents of this book or anything else with your physician. Most of the time your physician will actually be relieved to see that you are trying to do something to obtain excellent health and will encourage you to continue doing so. Never be afraid to consult your physician about anything that you feel is unusual or would warrant their attention. Most physicians will be excited that you are trying to improve yourself and will definitely want to keep a close eye on you medically and especially if you currently take any prescription medications that are necessary due to previous dietary indiscretions.

As you repair your health, your medication needs will decrease or be significantly altered, and you will need to have a close working relationship with a knowledgeable physician who will be interested in watching you make excellent progress. Your physician will need to adjust your medications as needed.

Never underestimate the power of a good and healthy diet in restoring your health. A rapid decrease in the amount and type of medication that is required to treat common chronic illnesses is expected with an excellent diet. If you are taking prescription medications or have already been diagnosed with any medical condition, make sure that your physician is aware of your eating plans and that you will likely need to have your medications adjusted accordingly. A change in medication levels will likely be needed after just a week or so of eating a healthful diet and then again after another week or so and then at a month out, again at three months out and again at six months out. Please work closely with your physician to be sure you do not make yourself ill by taking medication that was designed to maintain you on your traditional American diet. I cannot stress this enough. You must closely monitor your medications as your dosages are guaranteed to change in a short period of time.

When my husband first started eating healthfully, he suffered a pretty significant gout attack. This was likely caused by the excess body fat rapidly entering his blood stream due to the melting of his bodies fat stores. He went to see his physician, who was astounded to see how much weight he had lost in such a short period of time.

He asked his doctor if he should try to stop losing weight so rapidly as it was causing him to suffer from a gout attack. His physician replied that he could give him medication to manage the symptoms of gout but that if he had figured out a healthy way to get the excess weight off and keep it off that the weight loss would solve most of his health problems and he should continue doing what he was doing. He stated that getting people to lose weight is the most difficult part of his medical practice.

The expected side effects of eating healthfully are a normalization of blood pressure, blood glucose, weight and cholesterol levels as well as a normalization of heart rate. These results are typical and expected and only do not occur if the plan is not followed.

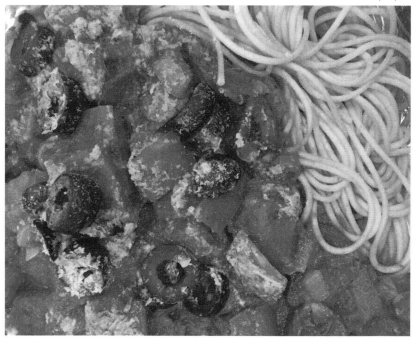

Chapter 3: The Truth About Carbs

Explaining Why The Ideal Human Diet Is Supposed
To Be Almost All Carbs And How None Of Those
Carbs Should Be "Candy" Carbs

When I was in school taking an exercise physiology
class, one of the first things we learned was that body fat
burns in a carbohydrate flame. What does this mean? It
means that in order for the body to most efficiently utilize
stored fat as a source of energy, (like when you are
exercising for longer than twenty minutes) carbohydrates

95

must be present in the diet. Think of the carbohydrates, or sugar, as kindling, to help get the fire going. If there are no carbohydrates in the diet, and carbohydrates are essential for brain and body function, what is the body to do? It has no choice but to break down muscle (the body's store of protein) so that it can use the sugar stored within the muscle tissue to help burn the fat and turn it into fuel.

Fat cannot be burned without sugar, which is most usually and most easily obtained from carbohydrates in the diet. The body can extract the carbohydrate from the muscle through a complicated process but only does this when it is in "starvation mode". The body only does this when absolutely necessary and as a result of this muscle breakdown, metabolic byproducts called ketones are produced.

These ketones are the byproduct of the body burning muscle, fat and fatty acids for kindling prior to utilizing the fat for fuel instead of burning its easiest source of energy, which are carbohydrates. These ketones that are produced can be easily measured in the urine. The body naturally tries to spare the muscle tissue from consumption until it becomes absolutely essential to use it. The popular Adkins diet, Wheat Belly Diet, Zone Diet, Sugarbusters Diet, Paleo Diet, ketogenic diet or whatever the new name is for the diet in which people eat a nearly all protein and fat diet, and avoiding almost all carbohydrates, is physically hard on the body.

If you deprive monkeys of their fruit, what happens? When you look at the people who eat this way, do they glow with health? Are they animated and energetic? Are their eyes bright and shiny? Is there skin softly pink? Do they appear to be fit and healthy? No, they do not. They appear sallow with a funny texture to their skin, have terrible breath and often body odor, and often likely have the beginning of kidney problems from ingesting too much protein in their diet. Tests for kidney disease administered at your physician's office do not show signs of kidney damage until the kidney's function has been decreased or compromised by eighty percent or more.

People eating this kind of low carbohydrate, high fat diet frequently experience heart palpitations, dizziness and often suffer from chronic constipation. This being said, their cholesterol levels are fairly normal, according to the current American standard of two hundred or less. Of course this doesn't mean much as research has shown that a cholesterol level of below one hundred fifty is truly needed to prevent heart disease.

Ketone bodies present in their urine is a sign that something in the body is malfunctioning and is not working normally. People on low carb diets, Type I diabetics and people suffering from the disease anorexia nervosa and those who are in the process of starving to death usually produce ketone bodies in their urine. Ketone bodies are not found in healthy people, they are found in ill people.

When a person uses a low carb diet, the body is tricked into burning all of its resources to try and protect life itself. This is what happens when the body is pushed into its basic survival mechanisms. Dr. Robert Adkins plan was to initially have people eat no more than twenty grams of carbohydrate per day until they were in a state of ketosis. They were able to tell if they were in ketosis by using easily and widely available urine dip sticks to measure the ketones present in their urine. They were to stay in this state of ketosis until they had lost all of the weight that they needed to. After they had lost all of the weight that they cared to lose, they were to begin adding small amounts of carbohydrate back into the diet and to continue checking their urine for the presence of ketones until they found how many grams of carbohydrate that they could eat before the starvation process was reversed.

Dr. Adkins wanted his patient's to stay right on the edge of producing ketone bodies and this would help them to continue the Adkins diet forever on a maintenance type plan. Even Dr. Robert Adkins himself, author of the famous Adkins diet that began the current low carb craze, acknowledged, prior to his death, in an interview with Dr. John McDougall, that an ideal diet would be based on vegetables, fruits and whole grains, but he said that with the enormous problem of obesity in America we were not starting at the beginning so we couldn't be idealists. He said that people would never be able to stop eating the rich foods and things they know they are not supposed to eat so it was easier to just let them eat the high protein fats and meats and trick their bodies into believing that they were starving by eliminating the ingestion of most carbohydrates. Dr. Adkins agreed that vegetables, fruits and whole grains were the healthiest diet but said people would never be able to eat healthfully with all of the unhealthy options so easily available to them.

I don't know what your experience has been watching people go through the Adkins or other low carbohydrate type diet, but mine has been that at first they begin the plan and are like religious zealots spouting anti carbohydrate rhetoric and avoiding any foods with carbs while indulging in such questionable substances as unlimited pork rinds and cheese.

After a few weeks, they are indeed thinner but they also look a little funny. A few months into this plan some of them are approaching normal weight, and some have even managed to obtain a "normal" weight. A few more months go by and they seem to be caving in and eating carbs again, especially on special occasions.

A few more months go by and they are the same size they were before they started their low carbohydrate plan. They still speak the anti-carbohydrate language and vow to "get back on the band wagon" as soon as the next holiday has passed, but they are no longer following the plan, that much is obvious. Let's think about this. Was Dr. Adkins able to attain and maintain a trim and healthy body by following his own plan?

Dr. Robert Adkins died from head trauma after he slipped and fell on an icy sidewalk at the age of seventy-two. Accounts of his weight at the time of his death show that he was 6 feet tall and he was reported to have weighed 258 pounds. This weight was taken after he had been treated in the intensive care unit for two weeks and had been suffering from massive organ failure. His family states that his kidneys shut down and his body ballooned considerably as a result of retained fluid. His family states that the organ failure caused his body to take on a tremendous amount of water weight while he was being treated in the ICU. His family insists he weighed around 195 pounds upon admission to the hospital and not the 258 pounds that is recorded on his autopsy records.

Most medical professionals find it hard to believe that Dr. Adkins' ICU physicians would allow him to balloon with nearly 60 pounds from fluid retention alone. It would appear from this information that Dr. Robert Adkins, author of the Adkins diet books, was not only overweight upon admission to the hospital before his death, but was actually obese, with a BMI of 35.0. Prior to this he had been diagnosed with cardiomyopathy and on autopsy it was revealed that he had suffered a previous heart attack as well.

So Dr. Adkins himself struggled with excessive weight and was not only overweight but obese at the time of his death.

So does the Adkins diet work? Yes it works. It will help you to lose weight but may not put you into the normal range for weight according to the BMI scale and is so difficult to follow long term that even the author of the plan was unable to stick with the plan and died obese with evidence of a previous heart attack.

Will the Adkins diet make you healthy? No, this is not a healthy way to lose weight. Is it harmful? Yes, it likely is. The cardiomyopathy and reported history of a heart attack that Dr. Adkins had suffered from are not signs of excellent health. It appears that he was suffering significantly from heart disease. The body doesn't usually respond well to being "tricked" for long periods of time and there are always consequences, such as cardiomyopathy, heart attacks and heart disease. Our bodies are too precious to play games with.

I believe that we can and should do better than this. If we take a look at the cultures of the world where the people were naturally slender, such as in Asia and India, what do the people who live there generally eat? That's right. They eat a diet that consists almost entirely of carbohydrates. Not refined or "candy" carbohydrates, except for their unfortunate use of white rice, but unrefined and unprocessed carbohydrates.

They mostly eat the kind of carbohydrates found in vegetables, fruits, beans and whole grains. They do eat a lot of refined white rice, to their detriment, but overall they are much thinner and healthier than we are. The people in these countries do not have desserts in the way that we westerners enjoy them, but instead often eat fruit for dessert. They eat meat and fish sparingly, a few times a month at most and almost never eat dairy products.

Unfortunately the traditional diets in these much healthier countries are now also changing. As these countries become wealthier, they are adopting a western, very unhealthy, diet, and the people in these countries are starting to suffer from all of the same diseases and pathological conditions that our nation has been suffering with for the last several years. Thankfully, very detailed research into their dietary patterns prior to these recent changes was done, especially in China, before commercial success began to change the traditional diets of millions of Chinese. In the book called "The China Study" written by Dr. T. Colin Campbell, it has been proven that the longest lived, healthiest people in the world ate a plant based diet consisting of mostly vegetables, fruits, and beans with a little bit of meat and dairy on the side, way off to the side, and usually reserved for festivals and holidays.

The people of Okinawa, Japan were known to be the longest living people on earth. In the traditional Okinawan diet each day, the average Okinawan would eat seven to ten servings of fruit and vegetables, seven servings of whole grains and two servings of tofu. Fish was eaten two to three times per month. The Okinawan people eating this traditional diet were thin, with no hypertension, Type II diabetes, and minimal cancer and had very little other chronic disease states even well into advanced old age. There was no need for nursing home care as they were able to care for themselves as they always had even into well advanced old age. Instead of eating rice, like the mainland Japanese people, they ate a great deal of purple sweet potatoes. Their diet was absolutely chock full of carbohydrates and little of anything else and yet they were free of diseases, were thin and robust and lived long and healthy lives.

The evidence is clear. This is not a genetic predisposition to live a long and healthy life. This is the effect of proper human nutrition. If one were to take one of these people out of Okinawa and plant them in the middle of an American city or town, assuming he or she would be fully integrated with the general population there, and then come back in twenty years to see how things were going, what would we find? We would likely find our poor immigrant, who once had full health and vigor, would likely be fat and sick and taking handfuls of pills every day just like every other American over the age of thirty. If we compared this person to their brothers and sisters who had remained in Okinawa and continued eating the traditional diet that represents very close to optimal human nutrition, our subject would be much sicker. This is not a genetic problem, this is a dietary problem.

Some people think that the reason that the Okinawans were so healthy is that they did not experience the mental stress that we do on a regular basis in this country. Somehow people believe that living in close community groups with strong social ties and regular meditation practices do a great deal more to advance human longevity than diet does. I think that the close social ties and meditation and mindfulness help a little, but only make up a small percentage of the health and longevity puzzle. I think that the theory of stress causing diseases is not true as Nathan Pritkin's research into this area showed that disease rates actually fell for people whose countries were ravaged during World War II.

Nathan Pritkin's research shows that the people were actually physically much healthier during the war years, during the times of rationing of meat, eggs, and other animal products, than they were before the war began and again after the war was over and the people returned home. After World War II there was a huge spike in death and chronic diseases that appears to be caused by a return to "normal" eating patterns with the regular consumption of meat, eggs and dairy products. A return to their usual diets led to an increase in heart disease and cancer.

The physical and psychological stress that these poor people must have been under during World War II had to have been tremendous. Whole families were disrupted for years at a time and yet the rates of chronic disease decreased significantly during these war years. If chronic diseases were caused and / or made worse by living under stressful conditions, then the people whose lives were disrupted by the war should have been sicker during the war years and returned to health when the war was over. Strangely enough the opposite actually occurred.

Conversely, the opposite is also true. A person with an idyllic living situation and a very pleasant home life still dies from heart disease and cancer despite their relatives begging them to stay. There is nothing sadder than a life cut short by preventable disease. We have all witnessed this very sad and completely unnecessary event.

I think that there is more than enough evidence to implicate that a return to a regular diet heavy in milk, eggs and meat caused the increase in disease following the return of the soldiers following World War II. As Dr. John McDougall often says, "It is the food".

Looking in the mirror and comparing us to our closest living relative, the chimpanzee, it is clear that the diet we are supposed to and made to consume is a vegan to near vegan diet made up of unprocessed and unrefined vegetables, fruits, beans and whole grains with very little of anything else.

The saliva in our mouths contains amylase, which is an enzyme present in the saliva of vegetarian animals that helps to break down the starch in the food that we are eating. Carnivorous animals do not have amylase in their saliva.

The teeth in our mouth and the way that our jaws move indicate that we are meant to grind our food. The canine teeth we have in the front of our mouths are nothing compared to the real canine teeth of real meat eating animals. Take a look inside of your dog or cats mouth and see what a real carnivorous animals teeth look like. Now THOSE are canines! And even the back teeth, the molars of dogs and cats, are shaped like knives, with serrated edges, to slice up and into the meat as it is quickly swallowed and consumed. The jaws of cats, dogs and other carnivorous animals close like scissors to chop meat while ours go back and forth to grind plant materials. Our molars and teeth are flat when compared to true carnivores.

We human beings can see well in color and prefer to eat sweet things more than anything else. This is so we can eat FRUIT! Not Fruitloops! Not gummy flavored fruit candies but actual REAL fruit. We are supposed to eat a diet that consists of almost nothing but whole, unrefined carbohydrates with little else. A diet made up of vegetables, fruits, whole grains, beans, nuts and seeds and almost nothing else.

Another strange phenomenon is that human beings are the only omnivorous animal on the entire planet whose male members have seminal vesicles. All other animals that have seminal vesicles are plant eaters and only plant eaters. So the question is, are the other animals supposed to eat meat or is it the humans who are doing something that their bodies are not designed to do?

The human being is a survivor. Surviving is not the same as thriving. In order to be our very best, healthiest selves, a very near vegan diet consisting of vegetables, fruits, whole grains, beans, nuts and seeds is optimal.

If everyone ate like this, medical care costs in this country would dwindle to almost nothing. The health of the country would markedly improve and productivity would tremendously increase as illness of almost any kind would be rare.

A really good question is that if our ideal diet is a near vegan one then why do we eat animal products and refined oils? I think the reason we eat them is because they are available to us. They used to be rare treats or sometimes necessary for our survival but are now every day staples. Human beings are more like rats, cockroaches and other scavengers in that we can survive on a diet that is made up of almost anything edible. Yes, it is true that we can survive on diets laden with milk, meat, processed garbage foods and fat, but ideally, for best health and longevity, we should eat a diet of mostly unprocessed carbohydrates, including vegetables, fruits, beans, whole grains, nuts and seeds. A low carbohydrate diet can make you lose weight but likely will not make you thin or healthy. When carbohydrates are severely restricted or eliminated from the diet, the body believes that it is in starvation mode and responds accordingly. Carbohydrates are the bodies preferred source of fuel. This is why endurance athletes "carb load" before long races, so that they will have a plentiful fuel supply during their sporting activities.

So why is everyone so afraid of eating carbohydrates? Why does everyone think that eating carbohydrates will make them fat and unhealthy? This is simply the power of the media and of wishful thinking that good health is as easy as avoiding carbohydrates.

Eating meat, milk, eggs, cheese, oil and processed foods is what will make you fat. Even if you are not fat on the outside, your arteries will clog with fat and you will have hypertension and heart disease and if you are genetically predisposed to cancer, you are creating a perfect environment for it to thrive.

You will not get fat and sick from eating fresh, whole, unrefined carbohydrates. Your arteries will remain clear of blockages on this type of plan. Even white potatoes are not unhealthy; it is what is put on the potatoes that make them a poorer food choice. A person could quite easily LIVE for months on end eating nothing except potatoes and would be fine. White potatoes even contain vitamin C! (Kon S. XXXV. The value of whole potato in human nutrition. Biochemical J 22:258-260, 1928.) The same cannot be said of any other type of food.

Eating a diet of nothing but meat and fat leads to severe osteoporosis, as was often seen in the native Inuit people in Alaska, who often exhibited severe effects of osteoporosis with large dowager humps in the cervical and thoracic spines of people in their thirties, so why do we think that this diet will make us healthy?. Why do we eat diets that are so heavily laden with meat, milk, eggs, cheese, yogurt and processed foods? The reason we do this is because everyone else is doing it and so it seems normal. These are the foods that are heavily advertised in the media.

Back in the 1950's everyone was smoking, so it was considered normal. Now we know that this is unhealthful. Twenty percent of Americans choose to continue this habit even though they know it is unhealthful as it is very addictive. I believe the same thing will happen when people realize that being skinny, fit, healthy and beautiful is as easy as eating delicious whole, unrefined carbohydrates all day every day. I believe twenty percent of people will continue to eat poorly, out of choice or because they are addicted, but the educated people and the people who really care about themselves and their loved ones will make better choices with the proper information.

According to the book, "The Blue Zones", the evidence is clear that the food that the longest lived and healthiest people in the world consume on a daily basis is unrefined carbohydrates with very little of anything else. This can leave no question as to what we as human beings are SUPPOSED to eat. We are designed for and are supposed to eat a diet made up of complex carbohydrates with very little animal protein or added fat. When this diet is consumed, our weight normalizes, blood sugar and hypertension issues are resolved and Type II diabetes is reversed. Many other diseases, especially autoimmune diseases, also markedly improve on this type of diet. This isn't really a diet, it is a LIVE IT!

I call it a LIVE IT because eating this way most of the time is what will make you healthy, with a great deal of energy and improved function for all of your daily activities. The big question we should ask ourselves is if this type of diet leads to improved health and normalization of weight, blood pressure and blood sugar then why aren't we already eating this way? That is a good question. The real question isn't why, it is why not?

Fruits, vegetables whole grains and beans are known as complex carbohydrates. They are not simple carbohydrates. All experts in the field of nutrition, no matter where they stand in regard to this topic, agree that simple carbohydrates, such as white sugar and white flour, should be avoided and even eliminated from a healthy human diet. Yet if American's are not eating meat, eggs and dairy, their next favorites are white sugar and white flour. Why is that? It is because as human beings we need carbohydrates as they are our primary form of fuel and therefore we crave them.

All that a food manufacturer has to do to make a fortune in this country is to make a food that is highly palatable by using and combining together large amounts of very inexpensive sugar, fat, salt and white or corn flour and we will buy these products, eat them regularly and crave them and feel that we absolutely need them. (Think about the very popular chocolate wafer with vanilla cream filled sandwich cookies and doughnuts covered in a sugary glaze and filled with custard pudding, cream filled pastries, and corn chips dusted with spices after being fried in oil.) All of the really popular junk food items, which are phenomenal best sellers, are composed almost entirely out of white flour, sugar, fat and highly processed corn products.

Our brains demand carbohydrates so that we can think properly. The fuel that feeds our brains and every other cell in our entire bodies is glucose which comes from the ingestion of carbohydrates. Our brain, which runs exclusively on glucose and cannot use any other fuel to work, uses twenty percent of the energy that our body produces just to think. Glucose, our primary fuel, is most easily obtained from the breakdown of carbohydrates. Our bodies need carbohydrates to work out and feel energized. Carbohydrates give us our energy and help us to think clearly.

Human beings have lived for millions of years in a state of constant and chronic deprivation of food. Gathering enough food, any kind of food that we could eat, was essential for our survival. This activity naturally took almost all of our time and energy. Because of this constant hardship, our bodies are now hardwired to immediately be attracted to foods that are high in sugar, fat and salt, as these foods were the most valuable in times of starvation and illness.

For our ancestors, foods high in fat, sugar and salt very likely played a large role in the natural selection process that brought us here today. The person who could eat the most of these rare and highly palatable foods would out survive the rest, therefore living long enough to reproduce and pass on their genes. This is pure Darwinism. With that being said, in nature, foods that have an excessively high amount of sugar, fat and salt just don't exist. There is no way that our ancient relatives could eat excessive amounts of sugar, even if they wanted to, unless they were lucky enough to be in a royal or ruling class that had access to refined foods. Eating a piece of pure sugar cane won't put as much sugar into your body at one time as eating a bag of gummy bears will. Fruit is the food that comes closest to being able to do this, but you cannot eat enough whole fresh fruit in one sitting that will give you a sugar rush like a candy bar will. There is no reason to be afraid of eating fruit. All fruits, except for pineapple and watermelon, are lower on the glycemic index and usually won't raise your blood sugar very much. Even diabetics can usually tolerate eating most fruits without difficulty.

It is no wonder that we crave the foods that we do. Our brains and bodies are simply hardwired to want them and to find them to be the most valuable. But thankfully, now that food is relatively plentiful for many of us, this same mechanism that was meant for our survival has become detrimental to our good health. The natural inclination that we have is to survive by eating as much as we can of highly palatable foods, foods that contain unnatural amounts of sugar, fat and salt. Food manufacturers are aware of our weaknesses and continue to pump out enormous quantities of these cheaply made food items. We are hardwired to never turn it down and to seek it out and eat if first and because of the excessive quantities of these foods currently available in our society we are overloading our systems and causing disease's. Food that tastes this good are not natural and are not supposed to be so easily available. Food that is this easily obtained and this highly palatable has only become widely available in the last thirty years or so.

All carbohydrates supply the body with energy. Simple carbohydrates will supply energy, but at what cost? When simple sugars are consumed they are followed by increased sugar present in the blood. This causes the pancreas to immediately pump out insulin to help store the excessive sugar for later use in the muscles as glycogen. When the muscle stores are full, the rest is converted to fat and stored.

Excessive consumption of simple carbohydrates has also been shown to cause the body to have a feeling that most Americans equate with being hungry. A rumbling in the tummy is what most people associate with hunger. Like the feeling you get a few hours after eating Take Out Chinese Food, this rumble is thought to be the body asking for more food. People often experience rumbling in the tummy along with sweating and weakness and commonly call this feeling "hunger pain" or associate it with low blood sugar.

Most people believe that this feeling is caused by the blood sugar in their blood stream plummeting after a meal, indicating that it is now time for another meal. People even get somewhat cranky if they are not able to eat immediately when they began to experience this sensation.

Dr. Joel Fuhrman, author of several books on "Nutritarian" style eating, (the term nutritarian is his own word that he uses to describe his eating plan) has performed extensive studies on subjects and found that when the subjects are experiencing this tummy rumbling, their blood sugar is not really plummeting. Their blood sugar is, in fact, stable.

What Dr. Fuhrman believes this sensation is, and this makes perfect sense to me, is that this feeling is caused by the body going into a "housecleaning" or detoxification mode to rid itself of the toxic effects of the simple carbohydrates and garbage foods that have just been consumed earlier.

Yep, that's right. You heard that correctly. Basically everyone is a junk food addict and goes through "withdrawal" from their junk food every four to six hours or so and requires another "fix" of junk food to keep these withdrawal symptoms at bay.

Because Americans eat so much junk food and experience this sensation on a regular basis, we tend to associate this feeling with low blood sugar or hypoglycemia and as a result, we think we are hungry. Everyone I know actually thinks that this is a normal sensation. There is stomach cramping, gurgling and a feeling of weakness and shakiness that most people refer to as "hunger pain".

My young nephew, at the age of seven, was running around in circles with his hands over his stomach screaming about how hungry he was as he recently experienced this phenomenon while waiting for his lunch to be served. He was experiencing what Dr. Joel Fuhrman, in his book "Eat to Live" describes as "toxic hunger". This is not what real hunger feels like.

Dr. Fuhrman states in his book that most Americans have never experienced real hunger. He describes the feeling of toxic hunger as a similar sensation to what the body goes through every time a noxious and addictive stimulus is removed. For example a person who drinks too much alcohol and then tries to stop it will go through a period of detoxification in which they will feel ill, they will have stomach cramps, they will sweat and they will be nauseated. To stop this process and put an end to the detoxification process, they can drink more alcohol. That doesn't solve the problem; it simply puts the detoxification process off for another day.

The process of detoxification must still be gone through if a person wants to be free of an addiction. A person who smokes cigarettes has also experienced this phenomenon. The first cigarette ever smoked is toxic. The body fights its ingestion with coughing and sneezing, letting the person smoking know that this is not healthy. Instead of heeding the warning, a smoker will continue to smoke and soon the body stops giving warnings that this is noxious. But if that same person were to stop smoking, the body immediately begins to repair the damage and the person will actually begin to feel ill as a result of the clearing and detoxification process. Increased inflammation, headaches, fatigue and nausea will result. This ill feeling will not usually last more than a few days and is a necessary part of the healing process.

The same thing can happen when a person tries to decrease their dependence on caffeine. If a person drinks caffeine every day in the form of sodas or in coffee or tea and then stops, they will experience caffeine withdrawal in the form of a massive headache, shaking and weakness and possibly with sweating and nausea as well. This is the body's natural reaction when a noxious and addictive stimulus is removed and the healing process has begun.

This same sensation happens to people who stop eating simple carbohydrates and junk food. Their body will feel ill as it begins the repair process. They will be dizzy and feel weak and they may sweat and have stomach cramps and gurgling. They may become irritable and cranky. The way to stop this feeling is to give in and eat some junk foods and simple carbohydrates. But this means that the process will have to be restarted. When a person stops eating this junk, this ill feeling will disappear in less than three days in the case of toxic hunger and will only reappear again when simple carbohydrates or junk foods are again ingested, but this feeling will never be as strong as it was for that first three days.

Dr. Joel Fuhrman's description of the process is very interesting and a phenomenon that almost everyone, especially those eating the traditional or standard highly toxic and low nutrient American Diet can relate to. He states that when the body is given toxic food to eat, such as the simple carbohydrates in white sugar and white flour, the body responds to the "emergency" created by this influx like it would to any assault, such as cigarette smoke or alcohol. The stomach gurgling feeling that most people equate with being hungry is actually the body beginning its cleanup of the latest toxic substance ingestion. If these toxic items are never ingested, the stomach cramping with sweating and dizziness will never occur.

Eating fruits, vegetables, beans, whole grains, nuts and seeds does not lead to this feeling. The person eating mostly these healthy foods will not experience this feeling that most Americans call "hunger" as this is not real hunger but just the body's reaction to coming down from the "high" after junk food ingestion. This feeling that most people think and describe as "hunger" is really just detoxification from an addictive substance.

So what does normal hunger feel like? If several hours go by, the person eating a healthy diet will still not experience "hunger" pain. Instead they will just be overwhelmed by the sensation of wanting to get something to eat. The sensation of hunger will be in their mouth and throat. This sensation of just wanting to eat is "true hunger", a sensation that most American's have never experienced.

Complex carbohydrates give energy, health and vitality and they are the basis of a lifestyle diet that you can really live with. Eating a diet made up of almost all complex carbohydrates will make you skinny, healthy and give you a great deal of constant energy. I want to be perfectly clear on this point. There is no such thing as eating too much produce, including vegetables, fruits, whole grains and beans. I have come across several diet plans that attempt to limit the eating of extremely nutritious fruits and beans. All of us should focus on eliminating the foods that are unhealthy, such as soda's, cakes and cookies and pastries as well as fats and oils, and not attempt to limit the consumption of very nutritious fruits, vegetables and beans.

Fruits contain many antioxidants and phytochemicals that cannot be obtained in any other way except by eating them. With that being said it is possible to obtain too many calories and become or remain overweight by eating too many nuts, seeds, tofu and / or avocados and by drinking fruit or vegetable juice. It is possible to become heavy eating highly processed crackers and cereals, even those that claim to be made of "whole grains".

Drinking juice, even "green" juice, will not make you skinny. This is why. When you are hungry, your body sends out a signal to your brain saying, "We are low on Vitamins A and C. Go get some". So your brain receives a signal to start eating.

We are creatures of habit so you just eat the same stuff that you always eat which doesn't contain any vitamins (just read the label. There is next to no nutritional value in most of the commonly eaten foods). So the stomach processes the food and again sends the signal. Not enough vitamin C or A. Get some more. So your brain tells your body to keep on eating and again, no real nutrients are obtained. This continues day after day and month after month. You never lack for calories, in fact by now you are overweight or obese, but you never get the nutritional requirements met, ever. So you take a multivitamin. The body says, "Oh, wow. It's that stuff I have been wanting and needing. Too bad it is in a package I don't understand."

The multivitamin gets flushed out by the kidneys.

Then you start juicing. The body says, "Wow! This is just what I needed!"

And as a result you start looking healthier. Your skin glows. Your eyes are shiny. But because you didn't consume the necessary fiber, you don't feel full so you continue eating too much and as a result you don't lose very much body fat. So you are healthier because you are now getting many more of the essential nutrients that the body requires, but because juicing removes the fiber, without the fiber to fill up your stomach, you are still fat.

The only way to get REALLY healthy and thin is through a combination of proper exercise and proper diet with diet accounting for eighty percent of the plan and exercise the other twenty percent. No starvation is required. Starvation and discomfort from hunger should never be a problem when you are eating properly. EAT if you are hungry. This plan is about really listening to your body and getting back in touch with what it is telling you.

Let me repeat that juicing fruits and vegetables works well to increase the level of micronutrients and phytochemicals in the body that are so desperately depleted in most American's and other westerners, but it does not work in the long run and will not make you thin. When you take the whole fruit or vegetable out of its "packaging", you lose the essential fiber, and THE FIBER IS THE MAGIC. It really is.

The more fiber from whole plant foods that you eat, the fuller you will feel, the more satisfied you will be and the healthier and skinnier you will be. It is as simple as that. The only way to get REALLY healthy and thin is through a combination of proper diet with some exercise.

Eating a diet composed almost one hundred percent complex carbohydrates will not only make you skinny, it will make you amazingly healthy as well. It is not dangerous to eat this way; it is what you are SUPPOSED to eat as a very fancy and complex primate. Can you survive on meat, cheese and eggs? Yes you can. You can survive eating animal products but you will not thrive or be at your healthiest when eating animal products. Eating a proper diet made up of complex carbohydrates with no added oil and minimal to no animal products will make you skinny, fit, long-lived and healthy.

So to recap, the complex carbohydrates contained in vegetables, fruits, whole grains and beans are delicious, filling and essential for good health. The more of them you eat, the better you will feel. Avoiding refined sugar and refined grain products is absolutely necessary for maintaining good health and a slim waistline.

We are essentially very complex and sophisticated primates and complex carbohydrates should make up nearly all of our diet in order for us to be the healthiest people that we can be. What would you feed your favorite monkey? You would feed him bananas, oranges, apples, carrots, Romaine Lettuce, sunflower seeds, whole wheat bread and brown rice. In that way your monkey would be fit and healthy and live a long healthy life. Can you give your monkey meat, eggs and dairy? Yes, you can, but it should be in very limited quantities, a couple of ounces at the most and no more than one to two times per month, and used mostly to add flavor to the much more nutritious foods that he should be eating.

Do you need to feed your monkey meat, eggs or dairy? No, you do not need to feed him meat, eggs or dairy products and if you choose not to give these substances to your monkey he will be even healthier than all of the other monkeys.

What if someone is mad at you because you won't give your monkey meat, eggs and dairy? This is a very real problem. People can be just ridiculous and have very strong opinions about health and nutrition. They may accuse you of monkey abuse. Have them read this book so that they can better understand how unhealthy eating these substances can be. Should you ever feed yourself or your monkey simple carbohydrates? No, but it is human (and monkey) nature to do what isn't good for us sometimes and you should be aware that when you do make poorer food choices you will likely suffer from stomach cramping and gurgling with dizziness, unusual fatigue, sweating and nausea as the body goes through a detoxification process after their consumption and in the process of cleaning up after them. This does not mean that you are hungry, it means you are suffering and sick from eating JUNK! So stop eating junk!

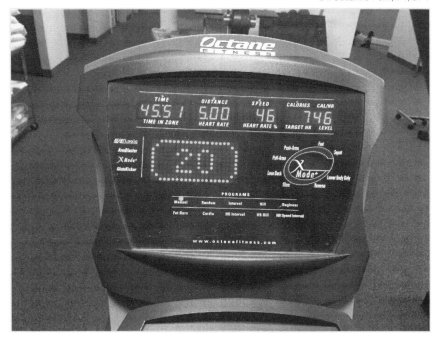

Chapter 4: The Truth About Exercise:

How To Perform A Fitness Self Assessment And What A Proper Exercise Program Looks And Feels Like

"Fitness is not what you sometimes do. It is WHO you ARE."

Lauren Kessler in the book Counterclockwise.

A good diet will make you look good in your clothes; exercise will make you look good when you're naked.

I am a physical therapist by profession. This means that I have a doctorate degree in human function and exercise and that I spend my days treating patients with exercise, modalities and manual therapy treatments to decrease their pain, improve their function and help them to return to their usual activities. To do this, I look at them, listen to them, measure them and then figure out what is missing that distinguishes them from others who do not have their particular dysfunction. Then I design a plan to get them from a place of dysfunction to restored function so that they can resume their normal activities without pain.

In my practice I have had so many clients and patients ask me how they can make their "six pack" abs show up or how they can get rid of excess fat on their upper arms. They tell me that they do so many sit ups and work out regularly but they still have belly fat and flabby arms. The reason for this is because they simply have too much body fat. You cannot see the muscles underneath the fat because they are covered with a layer of fat.

Dr. John McDougall has often said, "The fat you eat is the fat you wear". Fat that is eaten is very easily converted from your food to the fat that you then have on your body, requiring only three calories worth of energy to make this conversion from being the fat on your plate and on your fork into being the fat on your belly, thighs and upper arms. That means that ninety seven of every one hundred fat calories that you eat, beyond the amount of calories needed for your body to function, will be worn on your body for everyone to see. Fat that you eat changes its composition so little that according to Dr. Joel Fuhrman in his book "Eat to Live" he states that scientists can actually take a sample of your body fat with a needle, analyze it, and figure out the source of the fat. Even after being on your body the fat will still have the chemical composition of a pig, an egg, butter, vegetable oil, etc. If that doesn't disgust you, I don't know what will.

For the purpose of getting skinny and fit, I cannot emphasize this enough. All of the exercise in the world will not make you skinny and fit if you continue to eat a bunch of garbage. I have had so many athletic patients and clients that work out really hard and remain overweight and even obese. I have seen plenty of people running well in half marathons who are still significantly overweight and many who are obese. To be able to run these races and keep up the pace that they are able to, they had to have trained often and for long periods of time. If exercise alone could make you skinny and fit then these people would be skinny and fit. If exercise alone could make you skinny and fit then they wouldn't have to sell extra-large half marathon and marathon T-shirts, because nobody who could complete a half marathon or marathon would fit into them or need the size extra-large! It is very unlikely that anybody would be that big after all of that training. The sad truth is that exercise alone will not make you skinny. It isn't even half of the picture. It is only about twenty percent of the picture. Is exercise necessary? Yes, exercise is necessary. Regular exercise is an important component of a healthy lifestyle. I don't believe that you can be a really healthy person and not participate regularly in some type of exercise. It doesn't have to be terribly strenuous, but it does have to be regular and the more regularly you participate in it, the better you will look and feel.

I must be very clear on this point. You absolutely must change your diet in order to obtain good results and become skinny and fit. Exercise alone will not do it. This is especially true if you are over thirty years old. I think it is very necessary to emphasize again that successfully being skinny and fit is eighty percent diet and only twenty percent exercise. Exercise alone is not going to be enough to make you skinny or keep you there.

The "Lets Move" campaign, put together by First Lady Michelle Obama and the White House was a noble attempt at working in our schools to try and get kids running and exercising more but that is not going to make the school children thinner. Moving more will help a little bit, twenty percent worth, but increased exercise does not even cover half of this problem. Like Dr. John McDougall says, and I firmly believe, "It's the Food."

This chapter will have general guidelines that will assist you in taking a basic look at your general fitness and conditioning level. I will try to help you perform a physical self- assessment. With that being said, if you have any history of medical problems, if you are over the age of thirty or if you are very overweight or very de-conditioned, please check with your physician prior to making a self-assessment to be sure that you are fit enough to tolerate exercise. Consider asking your physician for a referral to a good physical therapist for an assessment of your fitness and general level of strength and conditioning. Many states have direct access laws in place that allow you to go directly to a physical therapist and undergo a physical fitness assessment and receive advice on what types of exercises you should do to increase your fitness and help to repair any deficits that are found with the evaluation that the physical therapist can see. I believe that physical therapists are the real experts in physical fitness assessments and are very underutilized in this country in this capacity at this time.

Exercise is a necessary part of living a healthy lifestyle. You have to exercise on a regular basis. It is healthy and good for you to do so. Exercise does not have to take a lot of time. I believe that most people can do very well with a healthy diet ninety seven percent of the time and three to five hours a week of exercise. Yes. You read that right. It only takes three to five hours a week of regular exercise to be skinny, fit and beautiful.

The US Government recommendations state that you need one hundred fifty minutes a week or two and a half hours. I personally think just a little more is necessary, with one hundred eighty to three hundred minutes a week or three to five hours. The good news is that this means you can skip days. That means you do not have to devote

yourself fanatically to exercise as a religion in order to look like a million bucks. It only requires three to five hours a week. I know you are busy, we all are, but finding three to five hours of week to take care of the one thing in this world that takes care of you is not asking too much.

One of my favorite cartoons depicts a patient standing next to a doctor's exam table with the doctor standing in front of him and the doctor is asking the patient, "What fits your busy schedule better, exercising one hour a day or being dead twenty four hours a day?"

This cartoon sums up my feelings about exercise. I do not believe that you must exercise for one hour every day, but three to five hours a week is necessary.

It really is ridiculous to think that we cram our lives so full of things that must be done that we don't even have time for one hour of exercise a few days a week. All of us are given the same one hundred sixty eight hours a week to divide the best that we can. You only need three hours out of the one hundred sixty eight hours per week to make a huge impact on how you look, feel and sleep at night. Three hours out of one hundred sixty eight is 1.7 percent of your week that needs to be devoted to exercise. This is less than two percent of your allotted weekly time. I don't care how busy you are, all of us can find three hours a week to take care of our bodies. Without our bodies we literally wouldn't have a place to live. Three hours a week of maintenance has to be done and we all have to find a way to fit this into the schedule. Exercise is essential for good health and for good body maintenance. It doesn't have to be that difficult to do. Simply making the commitment to do it and then showing up, even when you don't feel like it, is all that is necessary.

Once you get started, you might as well keep going. It is up to you how often you do it. My personal philosophy is that once I am sweating, I might as well keep going. What I mean by this is that once I have already made the commitment and put on the gym clothes and laced up the sneakers, once the first drop of perspiration falls, I might as well just keep going. I have no trouble showing up to exercise, properly equipped and ready to go. I have no trouble getting started. With that being said, about fifteen to twenty minutes into the exercise session I am no longer happy to be there and I have had enough and I would really like to quit except that I am supposed to keep going. It is a mental battle for me from the twenty minute point on until around the forty minute point and after that that I really don't care anymore and my energy picks up and I could literally continue exercising for a very long time. That is how my exercise routine usually goes. My husband, on the other hand, hates to get started. He will put off getting started as long as possible but once he gets going he can literally keep going, getting more and more motivated to continue, for hours. Everyone will be a little bit different.

I personally like to exercise for one and a half hours three days a week. That makes it a total of four and a half to five hours a week or so. I will just do the ninety minutes of exercise a few times a week instead of the one hour of exercise every day five days a week. Every person is different. To fit this into my life, after work, on Monday's and Wednesday's, I immediately change into exercise clothes and get started with my exercise routine. Then on the weekends, either Friday night, or some time on Saturday or Sunday I will exercise as well.

I only very rarely exercise in the morning before I go to work. It just doesn't feel right to me. I know that most people like to exercise in the morning and that is absolutely fine. I find it easier to exercise in the morning on the weekends. The timing of the exercise does not really matter, it only matters that it gets done. I know many people like to exercise early in the morning so that it will be done for the day and I know there is some controversy about exercising later in the day, but my personal philosophy is to just get it done whenever there is time to do it and to not worry about the timing so much. When it is done, it is done. Exercise can be a lot like saving money for retirement. There are a lot of different theories and people can spend hours and hours debating the subtle nuances that lead to supposedly better strategies and different outcomes, but the reality is that ninety seven percent of both exercising and saving money happens by just doing it.

As I mentioned earlier, my husband is a reluctant exercise starter. If he gets home from work and sits down in front of the TV, it is over. He will not be able to change gears and begin exercising. It is safer to just drop him off on the way home from work so that he can run the last three miles or so back to the house so that he will be done with the aerobic fitness portion of exercising before he even hits the front door. Once he is in the exercise mode he will keep on going, so when he gets home after running, it doesn't bother him at all to do twenty or more minutes of strength training and then some stretching exercise.

The important thing to keep in mind is that everyone's approach to this will be different. Once my husband gets started exercising, he never looks back. He just pushes himself for the entire time he is exercising. It is not the same for me. It is easy to get me started with exercise but then I require a lot of encouragement to keep going. Just remember that everyone is different. You will need to find your own style and do what works the best for you.

For some people it is much easier to commit to regular exercise with a buddy or two than it is to go at it alone. If you can get a group of three people it is even better because if one of the group members turns wishy washy and has family problems, commitment issues and a bunch of sick days, there are still the two of you together. Bigger groups are even more fun but it is important to maintain a personal connection within them so that you feel like your presence within the group really matters.

Some people just like to and are only able to commit to exercising alone. I like an exercise partner myself but because of my schedule it is difficult to find anyone who wants to exercise when I am available and it is hard for me to exercise on someone else's schedule. The important part is that because I know it is absolutely necessary and very important I will do it alone if I need to. The important thing to keep in mind is that nobody ever finished exercising and then said they wished they had not done it. It always makes you feel great and the best part of all is being finished.

"But wait", I can almost hear you say,

"Won't eating a diet made up primarily of plant foods limit the amount of protein available in my body to build and maintain muscle mass?"

After all, everyone knows that you need a lot of protein to build big strong muscles. Actually, this is not true. Eating plant based proteins, like broccoli, romaine lettuce, kale, whole grains and beans will provide not only adequate protein to feed your growing muscle mass, but the protein will be made up appropriately so that the muscles can actually be seen instead of being hidden under a bulky layer of excess fat. The whole food carbohydrates provided by a proper diet will give the exercising person plenty of energy to participate in regular physical exercise and the diet described in this book contains plenty of protein to build more than adequate and shapely muscle mass on both men and women.

Usually building muscle comes down to hard enough workouts and an adequate calorie intake. Taking in enough calories is not usually a problem as exercise leads to an increased appetite which leads to a natural increase in calories taken in. So do not worry that you are not eating enough protein ever. With adequate whole food calories you are getting plenty of protein and will build your beautiful, fit body with the plant based proteins. You do not need to supplement with protein powders or shakes or "muscle milks". These are unnecessary and a waste of money. You do not need to worry about eating the proper combinations of food to build complete proteins. Again think of a gorilla. He has a huge muscle mass and is very strong on a green protein diet. If you are really worried about it just perform a quick internet search for vegan weight lifters or vegan athletes and note that they all look very healthy and fit. They are definitely not suffering from a lack of protein and you won't be either.

Types of Exercise

This brings us to the types of exercise. There are three main types of exercise. First there is exercise to improve your endurance and cardiovascular function, also known as aerobic type exercise, then there is strength training to improve your muscular strength and then there is stretching to help improve your flexibility. All three of these components need to be incorporated into your exercise plan in order for you to be truly fit.

I know many runners who have excellent cardiovascular endurance but do not stretch or perform strengthening exercises and are prone to injuries as a result. I know many weight lifters who have excellent strength but who do not stretch or perform aerobic conditioning exercises, again leaving them prone to injury. I know many yoga enthusiasts who are very flexible but who do not strength train or perform aerobic conditioning exercises and are also prone to injury. All of these individuals are fitter than their friends who participate in no exercise, but they are missing entire components of real fitness. A really fit person will work components from each one of these items into a regular exercise and fitness program. A truly fit person will spend time working on each of these three types of exercise within every exercise session.

I am a runner. I am a reluctant runner. As a child I was not athletic in the least. I would rather read books than move around. I frequently suffered from neck and headache pain and general deconditioning. This persisted into young adulthood. I was brought up to believe that excessive exercise, which included most exercise, was bad and maybe even harmful to the body.

When I was eighteen years old I worked at a discount store similar to K-Mart in the Mid-West. I purchased an exercise bicycle at a deep discount when it went on clearance and set it in front of my television. I rode it for five miles and felt pretty good. I told my mother what I had done and she was very alarmed and begged me not to do it again as she was afraid that I would injure myself by riding a stationary bicycle more than just for short distances. She told me that I may damage myself with exercise and as a result I didn't ride that bicycle that far ever again. Looking back on this, it really seems ridiculous, but I am amazed by how many of my patients have similar anxieties about exercise and how these myths can persist and are pervasive in some cultures.

Women often worry that they will get overly developed muscles that will make their legs and arms bigger instead of smaller with strength training and many people are concerned that they will suffer permanent injuries if they attempt running. Men and women are afraid that pain symptoms that they are experiencing will be made worse instead of better with physical exercise. Of course none of that is true. You will not overdevelop your muscles with moderate amounts of exercise and you will almost always feel better with exercise instead of worse. Lifting heavy weights will only make your muscles huge if you have a good deal of testosterone running through you, and most ladies do not have enough testosterone to build a large muscles mass.

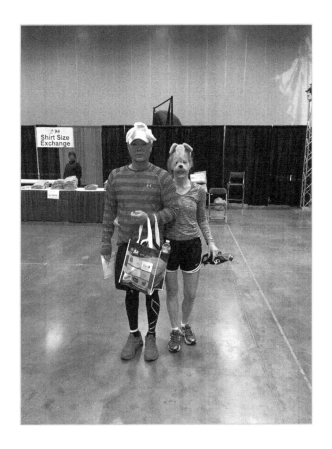

Aerobic Conditioning or Cardiovascular Exercise, aka Cardio

How good is your endurance? Do you get winded just climbing a flight of stairs? Could you go out for a half hour run? Aerobic conditioning is one of the easiest places to begin an exercise program because for many people just taking a walk will get them started. If you are over thirty years old and /or suffer from any medical condition, be sure to ask your physician's advice before beginning any aerobic conditioning or any other exercise plan. If you are relatively young and healthy, a good walk is the place to start.

Wearing comfortable shoes just open the door and walk away from the house for fifteen minutes and then walk back. Take the dog with you but don't let him walk you, you walk him, "Cesar Milan" style. That means the dog gets to do his business and then you get down to business with the dog walking beside you or slightly behind you and not dragging you all over the place and stopping to mark everything. You set the pace, not the dog.

If it has been a long time since you exercised it will be much easier on that first day than it will be for the next few weeks, so make it count. The next day, or the day after if you are a three day a week person, repeat the walk. It will surprisingly be more difficult. Your muscles may be sore from the first day and you will fatigue and think you can't do it, but you will finish and feel great. The third walk may be harder still. Keep going. The fourth will be tolerable, the fifth will start to feel annoying but neutral and the sixth will be almost as easy as it was the first time. Stick with it. Around the seventh, eighth or ninth time, depending on how good your general health is and how good you feel, increase either the time or the distance that you walk. A good rule of thumb is to add ten percent to either the time or the distance every couple of weeks. Then you just keep adding from there. Do not make the mistake of increasing exercise rapidly as this almost always leads to injury and then to rehabilitation of the injury which may derail your exercise plans completely.

Be sensible. Use a sensible approach to increasing exercise and be persistent. I like to spend somewhere between thirty and sixty minutes per session on aerobic conditioning type exercise. My family has a pretty good history of heart disease and I am doing my best to keep my arteries clean and flexible. I really don't enjoy running but I know it is very good for me and it is easy to do and so I do it. You can also go swimming if you are so inclined and have easy and regular access to a pool, or use an elliptical machine or a treadmill if you have access to these pieces of equipment.

It is even better for you if you switch up your activities on a regular basis. For instance I like to run but I try to use the elliptical trainer at least once a week to avoid any overuse injuries associated with just doing the same thing every time I exercise. If you have access to other forms of aerobic conditioning equipment, feel free to change the routine with every session. The important part is that the exercise gets done.

Using a regular stationary bicycle likely won't help to improve your cardiovascular fitness much unless you started out in a very de-conditioned state. If the exercise bicycle is all that you can manage, then it is better than nothing, but something a little harder to do would be better.

Whatever aerobic exercise you decide to do, it should feel a little bit annoying while you are doing it. Once your body is actively working, your mind will be working hard to come up with any excuse for stopping the exercise and it becomes a mental battle that you must learn to ignore, either by talking to others while exercising, paying attention to the scenery or the dog, or cell phone or by listening to your favorite upbeat music.

I have even figured out how to update my Facebook account while on an elliptical and for me this makes the time go by very quickly. You cannot allow your mind to make your body stop until it is time to do so. Figure out how much time you will be performing the aerobic conditioning exercise before you begin. Set the time that you will be working before you get started and stick to this time unless an actual injury takes place.

Usually, thirty, forty-five or sixty minutes should be the goal. Remember, aerobic exercise should be annoying but not unbearable. On a scale from one to ten it should be between a four and seven annoying. While you are participating in aerobic conditioning exercises it should be easy to talk but not easy to sing. If you cannot talk, you are exercising too hard. You will need to slow down a little until you can easily talk while exercising. If you can sing, you need to pick up the pace until you can talk but not sing Aerobic conditioning exercise is not only good for your heart; it is also good for your waistline.

If you eat a carbohydrate rich whole food, such as a banana, about a half hour prior to exercise and drink a glass or two of water you will create the perfect fat burning environment within your body. When you start an aerobic conditioning type exercise your body will start by burning the stored glycogen in your muscles for fuel over the first twenty minutes of exercise but after that, if you can talk but not sing, it is pure fat burning time from twenty minutes through the time when you finish the aerobic exercise session. So if you have a substantial amount of weight to lose, spending a lot of time in this special fat burning zone is an excellent idea and a great way to help the process along. Anywhere from thirty minutes to ninety minutes is perfectly fine as you work to increase your endurance.

With that being said, if you cannot even talk while performing aerobic conditioning exercises, you have entered the anaerobic phase of conditioning. This means that fat burning will slow as your body just tries to keep up and stay alive. You will increase your aerobic capacity and VO2 max with anaerobic intense exercise but for most people this is not necessary. (Definition of VO2 Max from the Merriam Webster Dictionary: The maximum amount of oxygen the body can use during a specified period of usually intense exercise that depends on body weight and the strength of the lungs. Also called maximal oxygen consumption). VO2 is a measurement of how good your body is at taking the oxygen from the air and putting it into the blood stream as efficiently as possible by going through the heart and lungs. It is essentially a measurement of cardiovascular fitness level.

For this reason it is better to spend a long amount of time performing a lower intensity aerobic conditioning exercise like walking, using the elliptical, running or swimming, than it is to rip and roar through a twenty minute high intensity exercise session at ninety miles per hour when you can't even catch your breath, let alone speak. Remember, the fat burning starts after the first twenty minutes of exercise. Until you hit that twenty minute mark, you are just burning the glycogen, or stored sugar, out of your muscles. If you want to burn body fat, then you have to continue working out past the twenty minute point on a regular basis in the aerobic fat burning zone, which means you can talk but you cannot sing. The longer time you spend in this zone, the more fat the body must burn for fuel.

Again I feel the need to emphasize that it is important to switch up your aerobic conditioning routine on a regular basis to avoid any repetitive use type injuries and to condition your body properly. My physical therapy clinic is full of athletes who exercise the same way, every time they work out and have become injured as a result. To avoid being a victim of a repetitive use injury, you have to vary your routine on a regular basis. In my case, I run a few times a week and then use the elliptical. I usually do one long session of aerobic conditioning, like a six to eight mile run, usually on the weekend. The other two exercise sessions will be shorter such as thirty to forty minutes long for the aerobic conditioning portion of the exercise. Remember, the goal is three to five hours of exercise per week split up however it is best and most convenient for you. Some people will thrive doing five shorter exercise sessions a week and others will do better with three longer sessions. You will need to get to know your own body and after some experimentation you will know what is best for you. The only thing that really matters is that you do the exercise and that you do it consistently.

So to recap, you need to do about thirty to ninety minutes of aerobic conditioning exercises, whatever kind you choose to do, three to five days a week.

It is important to do some cross training so that you will not suffer any overuse injuries. Cross training should be done at least once a week.

Again, you need to be able to talk but not sing while performing aerobic conditioning exercise. If you cannot talk you have entered the anaerobic phase and you need to slow down. If you can sing, you need to pick up the pace as you are not exercising hard enough to gain aerobic conditioning.

Remember that it takes at least twenty minutes of aerobic exercise to burn up the available glycogen in your muscles in order to begin burning fat for fuel, so if weight loss is your goal, you need to perform aerobic conditioning exercise for more than twenty minutes at a time.

Strength Training

Strength training is where many people get confused and there is a lot of misinformation. First things first, as a woman you will not overdevelop your leg or arm muscles with strength training unless you work extremely hard at it and you are naturally inclined to do so or you are a male with adequate testosterone. So many women are afraid of strength training as they are worried that their muscles will get too big and will be unattractive instead of more attractive. This is simply not true.

The average person working out three to five hours a week is not going to develop herculean muscles, especially if they are a woman. Women simply do not have the testosterone naturally present in their bodies that men do. Men do have plenty of testosterone, especially on a vegan diet, and will develop very nice bulk and definition in their muscles with regular strength training. Most women will just get arms like Michelle Obama or Jennifer Aniston who are both skinny and fit and beautiful.

Most people think that they have to buy expensive equipment to participate in strength training. This is simply not true. If you happen to belong to a gym, use it. The circuit training machines are easy to set up and you should run through them with three sets of ten to fifteen exercises two to three days a week. But do not despair if a gym membership is not available to you. Think about a prison inmate, locked in a cell twenty three hours a day. These prisoners are usually very fit if that is what they want to be and if they can do it, well then you can do it too. All you need is your body. Your body will provide you with plenty of resistance. Again, going back to childhood physical education classes, you can start very simply with pushups and sit-ups. If real pushups are too hard, start with pushups on the wall, then push-ups on a bench and finally pushups on the floor, first with your knees touching the floor and finally with your knees off of the floor. You can start with "girly" pushups and add real military style pushups on the floor when you are able to. Remember that you are only competing with yourself. Try not to compare your progress to anyone but you. This is not a competition.

When performing sit-ups, do not anchor your feet under anything and keep your knees bent up and your feet flat on the floor This helps to isolate the abdominal muscles as they like to hide and make the hip flexor muscles do all of their work whenever possible. Most Americans, especially those who sit at desks all day, already have very tight hip flexor muscles, and do not need to strengthen and tighten them any further.

Lunges are also easy to do as are standing squats. When performing squat or lunge exercises, make sure to squat back, like you are attempting to sit down in a chair, so that your knees always stay behind your toes. This will help you to avoid injury to your knees. If you are having difficulty with this, place a chair behind you and then squat, like you are about to sit on the chair, but come up before your behind actually makes contact with the chair. That is a proper squat form.

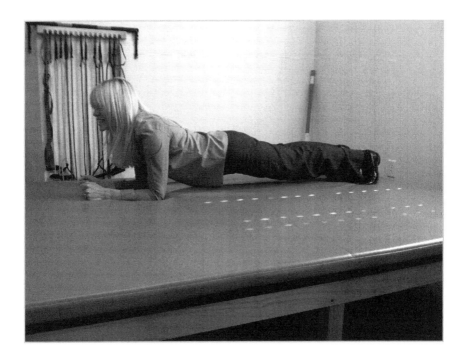

You can use your imagination and come up with all kinds of ways to strengthen your muscles. You can use pull up bars and other equipment for body weight resistance. Pay particularly close attention to core strengthening, using planks, side planks, sit ups, clams, straight leg raises, superman's, bird dogs, and push-ups of all kinds. The more time you spend developing your core muscles, the better off you will be and the more your athletic performance for all kinds of activities will improve, even going up and down stairs and carrying kids and groceries. The core muscles provide stability for all other exercises and for daily living activities. If you have a strong core, everything else gets easier, even running.

You should spend anywhere from ten to thirty minutes of your exercise sessions working on improving your strength. Use your imagination, the internet and You Tube and have fun doing it.

The saying, "No pain, no gain" originally developed for use with strength training exercises. Aerobic conditioning and stretching exercises can be slightly uncomfortable while being performed but the discomfort is usually over as soon as the exercise is. Muscle growth and strengthening is best obtained when the muscle is pushed hard enough that it starts to "burn" a little bit. Not a lot, just a little bit. The chemical explanation for this burning sensation is that the adenosine triphosphate, or ATP is being broken down into adenosine diphosphate, or ADP, within the muscle itself. The muscle running out of the ATP is what causes the burning sensation. This is your muscles message to your body that there is not enough strength in this location for what it is being asked to do. So when you are finished working out, your body assesses what happened and then adjusts its resources to address the apparent shortage that was there at the last strength training session that caused the burning sensation. The next time you perform the same routine, the body is better prepared with increased ATP available to fill the need and after a few sessions, you will need to increase the amount of weight that is lifted or you will increase the amount of repetitions that are done to produce that same "burn".

Notice that this is a mild "burning" sensation that is located in the body or middle of the muscle and not a "tearing" sensation. Do not ever exercise into pain that is more than this mild burn that occurs in the mid muscle area. To do so will actually cause you to be injured and then you will have to rehab the injured body part, which will interfere with your fitness goals. I tell my patient's that they should never experience pain that is more than a 3 - 4 out of 10 while exercising. If their pain goes over that, they must slow down or stop as they are doing more damage than good.

Traditionally, to gain muscle mass, you have to lift weights that you are able to lift no more than eight to ten times before you simply cannot lift the weight again. If you can lift the weight ten times, it is too easy for you to lift and will result in increased muscle tone but not increased muscle growth. If you would like the muscle to grow, the weight must be heavier. The weight has to be heavy enough that you cannot lift the weight more than nine times. After you lift the weight, wait a few minutes and attempt to lift the same weight another eight to ten times. Then you wait another few minutes and attempt to lift it a third time. If you are able to lift it for ten repetitions all three times, then the weight is too easy for you to lift. You will maintain the muscle mass that you have lifting smaller weights that you can lift for three sets of ten repetitions, but if your goal is to grow bigger muscles, you will have to make your body work for it. Of course if you are happy with your current muscle appearance, maintaining it with weights that you can lift ten times is fine. Again, keep in mind that it is important to perform a variety of strengthening exercises on a regular basis and to change your routine often to avoid repetitive use injuries.

Some people like to do a "leg day" then and "arm day" and then a "core day". You should try to incorporate strength training of your arms, chest, back, and legs into your training routine every week. Sometimes people make the mistake of only strength training their upper or lower body which leads to muscle imbalances. Another common problem is strength training only the front of the chest and arms and ignoring the back muscles. You have a whole body, use it.

Spend extra time on core strengthening as that is the most important strength exercises that there are. My sister hosted a ten your old Ukrainian orphan one summer and I was delighted and amazed to see how strong he was. His core strength was so good that he could squat down, and while maintaining his squatted position, jump up a flight of ten stairs without standing and without falling. He could do this repeatedly. He could do the most amazing stunts on the trampoline and could break dance beautifully. He could easily walk on his hands. This child had lived in an orphanage for several years with no access to a gym and very few toys but he was in excellent physical condition from simply being a child and exercising with what was available using only his body weight for resistance. If he can do it then so can you. Just put the time in to it, switch it up regularly, and keep on trying

So, to recap, you will not get giant muscles as a woman with resistance training. You will simply have very nice muscle tone. Men will grow large muscles because they have much more testosterone than women and that is what is needed to make muscles grow very large.

A very healthy whole food near vegan diet will provide you with all of the protein that you need to grow even large muscles without any difficulty whatsoever.

Resistance training will make you better at many of your usual activities, even climbing stairs, carrying books, groceries or children and almost all of your daily activities improve when your core muscles get stronger.

If you can lift a weight more than ten times it is not hard enough for you and you need to move up a level if your intention is to increase your muscle mass.

Do not ever exercise into pain but a small amount of muscle burning in the middle of the muscle belly is normal during strength training exercise as the chemical ATP in the muscle becomes depleted. It is not normal to feel ripping or tearing at the ends of the muscle and you should never exercise into that type of pain or you will do more harm than good. A good rule of thumb is that you should never experience any pain that you would rate as a 4/10 or higher while doing exercise. And of course, you should never take any kind of pain medicine or anti inflammatory drugs prior to exercise as you want to be able to feel what is going on inside of your body fully to prevent and avoid injury.

Flexibility

Can you bend down from the waist, and, while keeping your knees completely straight, touch your toes? You should be able to touch your toes at least with your fingertips. If you cannot, then either your back is inflexible or your hamstrings and or your calves are too tight and maybe even all of them are too tight. A few very flexible individuals will be able to do this and place their palms on the floor while keeping their knees straight, an obtainable goal for all of us to reach for.

Can you put your chin on your chest by looking down? Your chin should actually be touching your chest without any space. Can you put your head back and look straight up at the ceiling? Is it difficult to look behind you when you are backing the car up? If you cannot do these or have difficulty with them, then your neck is tight.

Can you reach your arms all the way up? If you try to do this and your arms are only part way up (look in the mirror), then your shoulders are tight. Lie down while looking at the ceiling on a flat surface and place your hands on the back of your head, lacing your fingers together. While doing this you should be able to squeeze your shoulder blades together and get your elbows very close to the surface you are lying on. You should be able to touch your elbows to the surface. If you cannot, you have shoulder and possibly neck tightness.

Can you reach with one arm behind your back and the other arm over the same side shoulder and grasp the fingers of both hands together while behind your back? If not, then your shoulders are too tight. You should be able to do this with both of your arms.

Lying flat on your back can you bend your knees and then pull your knees up all the way to your chest, in essence hugging your knees to your chest? Your knees should actually come in contact with your abdomen and chest. If you cannot do this then it is possible that your low back, your hips or your knees are too tight and maybe all of them are too tight.

Can you sit on the floor with your legs straight out in front of you comfortably without using your hands to brace yourself? Your legs and torso should be at a ninety degree angle. If you cannot keep your knees flat with your legs straight out in front of you and this is uncomfortable or impossible for you to do, your low back, your hips, your hamstrings or your knees are tight, and possibly all of them are too tight. From this "long sitting" position you should also be able to touch your fingertips to your toes. If not, then again, your low back, hips, hamstrings and / or calf muscles are likely too tight.

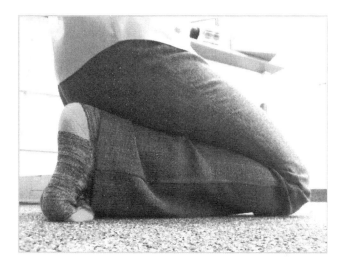

Can you kneel down on your knees, with your toes bent backwards (upwards) and pointing towards your knees and sit back on your ankles with your buttocks resting on the back of your heels? You should be able to do this easily.

If you cannot do this then your foot, quad muscles, calf muscles and you knee/ ankle/and or toe joints and possibly all of these are too tight.

Can you stand against a wall with your heels touching the baseboard, your behind touching the wall, your shoulders and the back of your head all touching the wall comfortably? There should be a gap of no more than two hand widths between your mid back and the wall if you are pretty thin. If the gap between your mid back is larger than two hand widths or you cannot touch the wall with your heels, buttocks, shoulders and back of the head all at the same time then you likely have poor posture.

Can you carry a medium sized hard covered book on top of your head without holding onto it while walking across a room? If not, you are probably looking down while you are walking, possibly with slouched shoulders.

While you are standing normally, have someone take a picture of you from the side. What do you see? Are you standing with good posture or is your head in front of your shoulders. Your head should be on top of your shoulders. Are your shoulders rounded or straight? Your shoulders should not be rounded forward. Is your pelvis straight up and down like a bowl? Or is it tilted forward or backwards? It should be straight, like a bowl, not tilted forward or backwards. Are you locking your knees backwards while you stand? Never, ever lock your knees. This can lead to arthritis. People do this because it is easier to stand for long periods of time and this position requires minimal energy to maintain but it is not good for your knees. Your pelvis should be a bowl, tilted neither forward nor back. Your knees should not be locked back while you stand. Your head should be directly on top of your shoulders. Your shoulders should be relaxed but upright and not tilted forward. If your head is in front of your shoulders and your shoulders are rounded forward instead of straight, you will need to work hard to correct your posture as this will eventually lead to neck and shoulder pain and dysfunction if it is not already causing pain. I always tell all of my patient's to put their chests out and their chins down. It feels strange at first but looks very nice and helps to correct posture.

To improve your flexibility you will need to stretch consistently. Some people find participating in a yoga or Pilates class a great way to get started with stretching and flexibility exercises. If participating in this type of class is not your style, then just regularly stretching after your workout for eight to ten minutes or so will really help.

Performing all of the usual stretches that you learned in elementary school physical education classes, like hamstring stretches, quad stretches, calf stretches, hip abduction stretches, etc. Gently stretch, holding each stretch for thirty seconds or so, repeating them three to five times for best effect. Do not bounce while stretching just hold the stretch gently but firmly. You should feel some tension but no pain. Remember to stretch your arms and your neck as well.

Many people feel that they just aren't flexible and will never be able to stretch. They state that they were born this way and will never be flexible no matter how much they stretch. This is simply not true. Genetics does play a role in how flexible our bodies can become but regular stretching is a very important component to making this possible. I always tell my patients who tell me the sad tale of how they have never been flexible and insist that it will be impossible to stretch them out or improve their flexibility, that if they were adopted into a family of circus performers when they were young, that this flexibility would be an important component of the family performing routine and the daily flexibility exercises they would be forced to do would definitely help them be a part of the family business. The point is that you are good at what you spend time doing. You may not ever be great but you can be good. If you never spend time stretching, you will never be flexible. It is as simple as that. If you take the time to stretch a few days a week, then your flexibility will improve. Spending the time doing it makes it happen

Many people ask when the best time to stretch is and the answer is at the end of your exercise routine. By then your muscles are completely warmed up and you have performed any strength training that you intend to do and it is a good time to stretch. Don't just limit stretching to exercise time, though. If you are sitting in front of a television and the commercials come on, take some time to stretch. If you are blow drying your hair in the morning, there is no reason why you cannot stretch your hamstrings at the same time. By incorporating stretching into our daily lives, it is easier to do and your flexibility will improve rapidly.

Many of my older patients are very inflexible and I believe that this lack of flexibility, coupled with an inflammation inducing diet are the leading causes of their pain. Working on and maintaining your flexibility is very important to your overall feeling of health and comfort as you age. As with anything, our bodies are programmed to "use or lose it". Very few of us were born being unable to turn our heads or bend down and touch our toes. It is simply a lack of use that leads us to this place. Maintaining flexibility is always better than working to improve it, but even when it is gone we can get it back with gentle stretching several times per week. We are living organisms and our bodies will adapt to our environment. Once good flexibility has been obtained, continue stretching on a regular basis so that your flexibility will be maintained.

If you are at a complete loss for a stretching routine, try this. First sit on the floor or mat table and spread your legs out as widely as they will comfortably go. Then reach to the right side, attempting to touch your right foot and hold three times for thirty seconds. Then reach to the center and hold three times for thirty seconds and then reach to the left side, attempting to touch the left foot and hold three times for thirty seconds.

After this, bring your legs together and reach down to try and touch your toes, holding three times for thirty seconds. Next, sit into a kneeling position with the toes facing the knees or bent up and the buttocks touching the backs of the heels and hold this position three times for thirty seconds. (Like the picture above). Then just change the position of the toes from pointing up, to pointing down and sit on the feet, holding this position three times for thirty seconds.

After this, lie on your back and pull your knees into your chest, holding this three times for thirty seconds. Then, keeping your knees bent up and your feet on the floor, lace your fingers together and place your hands behind your head and stretch your elbows back to touch the floor, holding this stretch three times for thirty seconds. Then, with your hands still behind your head, gently tuck your chin, making an ugly turkey neck and hold this stretch three times for thirty seconds. Then, reach your arms up high over your head and try to get them to touch the floor or surface behind you, gently stretching them and holding this three times for thirty seconds and then make some snow angels with your legs and arms a few times. There, stretching done!

So to recap, stretching is best done at the end of your regular exercise routine. You should spend eight to ten minutes stretching after working out and hold each stretch for thirty seconds performing them three to five times.

Incorporate stretching into your daily activities as well as being a part of your regular exercise routine. Even if you have never been flexible, you can work to improve your flexibility. Good flexibility will enhance your quality of life with less pain. This is especially true as you age.

It is important to note that exercise can lead to muscle soreness. As strange as it may sound, muscle soreness following exercise is very much improved and even minimized with proper nutrition. If you are eating the way this book describes, you will be amazed that you simply are not experiencing as much muscle soreness and general fatigue that you used to following participation in regular exercise. I don't' know if this is because the body is less acidic, I don't know if the chemicals and processed junk foods or excess sugar are to blame for the fatigue and muscle soreness that most people experience. I don't know if the excess animal based protein that most people eat is the main cause of excessive inflammation, soreness and fatigue following participation in exercise. I just know that with a proper diet you will have soaring energy, and when you do work out you will not have the usual muscle soreness that occurs with workouts.

Usually recovery from exercise should take less than forty eight hours with a proper diet. There will be some soreness but it will not be nearly as bad as what you have experienced in the past. If you do have some unusual soreness and fatigue, often times the best cure is to repeat the exercise that caused the soreness as this will help to pump blood into the sore and stiff muscle. Always remember to drink plenty of water as this will flush away any buildup of the products of muscle metabolism that may lead to or exacerbate this soreness and fatigue.

So, to summarize, no amount of exercise will make you skinny and fit if you eat a terrible diet. Exercise accounts for twenty percent of this plan while diet accounts for eighty percent.

It is very important to participate in exercise that lasts three to five hours every week. Nobody has this time available; we all must make sacrifices to care for our most precious possession, our bodies.

All three exercise components, aerobic conditioning, strengthening and flexibility exercises must be done every time you spend time exercising so that you will be a truly fit person and not prone to injuries.

Change or mix up or your exercise routine or cross train on a regular basis to avoid overuse injuries.

Be gentle but persistent with exercise and you will be rewarded with increased energy, less fatigue, and an increased ability to perform all of your daily activities. Pain during exercise is not normal and will lead to having to rehab injuries and might derail your fitness plans entirely. Slow and steady improvement is what we are looking for.

162

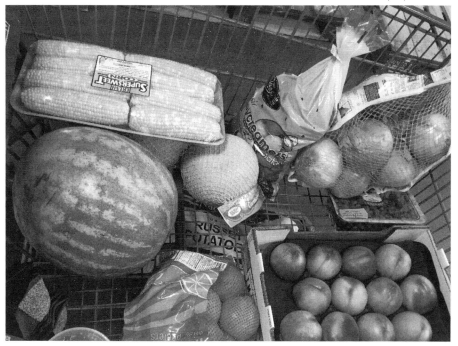

Chapter 5: The Grocery Store Is Where You Win The War:

What To Purchase And What To Leave Behind

There is a fountain of youth in every grocery store in the world and it is known as the produce department. Let me emphasize again that you cannot over eat produce. It simply isn't possible. As a very fancy primate, produce is your most important dietary staple. The United States government is recommending now that people eat nine servings of fruits and vegetables per day. The government's current dietary recommendation has increased from five

165

servings a few years ago. Produce takes up so much room in your stomach and intestinal tract that it is not possible to eat nine servings of produce at the same time that you are consuming a bunch of junk food. There is simply not enough room for the junk and the necessary amount of produce for proper nutrition.

If you eat junk food, you will blunt your natural appetite for produce. You cannot easily eat both junk and the amount of produce that you need. It just isn't possible. The truth is that most American's eat very little produce. They buy some and it is widely available for purchase in an astounding array of varieties, but they eat very little of it.

Most American's get forty or so percent of the calories in their diet from meat, eggs, and dairy products including milk, yogurt and cheese, an additional fifty or so percent of calories from highly processed, packaged junk food items and only seven percent of their daily calories from fruit and vegetables, with white potatoes, usually fried or mashed with unhealthy ingredients, making up four percent of the produce that is consumed. This means that for the average American, a diet that contains three percent fruits and vegetables is normal.

This lack of produce consumption is a serious health concern for both individuals and our nation as a whole. This lack of produce fills our hospitals with patient's suffering from chronic, preventable diseases and is in the process of ruining the financial health of our nation under the staggering weight of caring for these patient's through increased health insurance premiums and welfare to disabled individuals who are disabled because they eat nothing but junk all day every day and have become ill and unable to work as a result of this lifestyle. It is not their fault; they have simply not been educated and the junk food is highly advertised, very inexpensive and literally everywhere.

It is very important that we make significant changes in our country and start to really eat more produce as a nation. The fact that people do not know how important produce is for their health is because our country has a serious lack of basic nutritional education. People just do not know what proper nutrition is for a human being. When school children are young and studying nutrition, they are not told that they need to eat green leafy vegetables and whole pieces of fresh fruit every day. Instead, there is an emphasis on milk, so that they can obtain enough calcium, even though this overemphasis on calcium is completely unnecessary. There is an emphasis on eating animal products and meat. The children are told they need this for muscle growth and development. They are told that they must have protein rich foods in order to grow big, strong muscles. There is an emphasis on drinking bottled and likely unhealthy orange juice, so they will get enough vitamin C. There is no specific emphasis that they should eat broccoli, kale, romaine lettuce or spinach on a daily basis. There is no specific emphasis reminding them to eat fresh, whole apples, oranges, carrots and celery. The funny part is that you can easily, and more healthfully, live without milk, meat and orange juice, but your health will seriously suffer if you don't eat enough whole, fresh produce and especially green leafy vegetables.

It makes you wonder who writes this curriculum for the school systems and what their ulterior motives really are. Nutrition education really must change for the health of our nation. It is very important for all of us to eat leafy green vegetables and whole fresh fruit every day. This means that all of should be eating very large servings of spinach, kale, romaine lettuce, cabbage, Brussels sprouts and or broccoli at least once a day. This means that we all should eat three to four pieces of fruit every day. Just this act alone would make an enormous difference in the health of the people who make up our nation.

The battle of the bulge, the number on the scale, and for the most part the image that you see in the mirror are all determined and decided at your local grocery store. Most of us have schedules that are pretty tight and our schedules usually don't permit a lot of repeat grocery shopping for the week. This means that if you can make it out of the grocery store with only healthy, real food in your grocery cart you most likely won't have time to re-shop and ruin your best made plans.

I do most of my grocery shopping in the produce section of the grocery store. My cart is filled with bananas, apples, peaches, romaine lettuce, broccoli, carrots, mushrooms, white potatoes, sweet potatoes, spinach, corn, squash, lemons, green onions, cabbage, etc. It is important when you are shopping for groceries that you buy enough green leafy vegetable to eat them every day. The fresh ones are the best followed by frozen. Don't bother buying canned produce.

At the grocery store, there are the usual items that you purchase pretty much every time you go shopping. We all look forward to getting these comforting and familiar foods home and eating them. This has been a usual part of our routine for quite some time. Keep in mind that everyone has certain "trigger foods" that can cause you to have difficulty controlling how much you eat. For me, it is miniature peanut butter cups and any kind of white pasta product. Note that these items are considered junk food and are not permitted on a regular basis on this LIVE IT plan. If I start eating any one of these two items especially, it is very difficult for me to stop at what should be considered a reasonable portion size. Once you know what your trigger foods are, you should be careful to avoid them whenever possible. It is okay to enjoy these trigger foods once in a while as a special treat, but make sure you do so only when you know that the quantity will be very limited. For instance, I buy only whole grain pasta varieties. In the case of the peanut butter cups, I just don't have them around and I never buy them at a grocery store. If I go somewhere and they are available, for example in a candy dish at an office, I will eat only one or two on a very special occasion and then I will be done with it.

So, if your particular trigger food is something that is usually easily purchased at a grocery store, such as cookies, then do not buy them where you typically do and on those very special and rare occasions when you decide to indulge yourself with this trigger item, purchase it in a very small quantity, such as a single serve pack, from a convenience store or other place where you do not typically shop and purchase it at a different time then during your normal grocery run. Limit these types of purchases to no more than a few times per year. This is eating in true moderation.

The grocery store is where the real battle ground between healthy and unhealthy is fought. This is where the rubber meets the road. When you are putting this healthy diet plan into place, doing your best to make changes that you know will make you healthy, you must not put anything in your grocery cart that is not a part of this healthy eating plan. That means no chips, no frozen entrees, no ice cream, no white bread, no canned anything except for beans and some low salt tomato products, no oily salad dressings, no cooking oils of any kinds, no mayonnaise. No meat, no fish, no seafood. No butter, no milk, no eggs, no cheese. No yogurt, no fruit juice, no crackers, no rice cakes, no sweetened junky cereals and no white flour pretzels. And of course no candy and no white flour bagels! It is very important that you pay VERY close attention to what you place into your grocery cart. I cannot emphasize this enough.

You cannot bring home ANYTHING that is not a fruit, a vegetable, a whole grain low fat product, a bean, a nut or a seed for six whole weeks. That is because you are trying to change and if the stuff that you used to eat that made you fat and sick is in the house, it is just way too easy to get to it. It will be too easy to fall into the same habits that got you into the situation that you are currently in and therefore, at least for the first six weeks and possibly for a very long time afterwards and maybe even forever, it is important to not bring home from the grocery store anything that you are not supposed to eat.

If your household contains children, they should not have to ask for permission to eat anything because everything should be healthy and good for them and of course, they can have it. Let them eat whatever they like and whenever they like of whole, healthy, real foods.

Now that does not mean that you will never eat your usual favorite foods again. You may eat them in the future if you choose to do so. They will be there waiting for you at the grocery store. This is not forever, it is just six weeks, remember? So don't panic. You don't have to go all crazy eating buckets of junk in a "Mardi Gras" type show down on the day before the six weeks begins. That is just not necessary. You will be fine. It is only six weeks. I'm not saying that you should never again in your whole life eat meat, dairy, eggs or white grains, sugar, junk food and caffeine ever again. What I am saying is that the less you eat of these substances now and in the future, the younger you will look, the more energy you will have, the more muscle you will build and maintain, the stronger your bones will be and the less fat your body will store.

There is no question in my mind that the junk that you eat shows up on your body. It is something that can sometimes be hidden with clothing but it is always there. If you absolutely must have something that you are not supposed to have, then you must get into your car, drive to the place where this item can be obtained, buy it as a single serve item, eat it where you bought it, and come back home without it. Those are the rules.

So if you absolutely must have ice cream, get in your car, drive to Dairy Queen or wherever it is that you like to go and get some ice cream, and buy the smallest serving that they make, eat it and then come home without any extras. If you absolutely must eat some chips, go to the convenience store, buy one package that contains a single serving, and then eat this in your car, throw away the wrapper immediately and again drive back home without any extras. In this way you will seriously limit your intake of junk food as we are all way too lazy and have way too many other things to do than to drive around multiple times in a week in pursuit of one single serving of junk food. Do not ever buy junk food at your regular grocery store. Make sure that you have enough good to eat foods readily and easily available and when a craving hits, attempt to fill your stomach with as many allowed foods as possible in large enough quantities to alleviate the craving.

The real key to getting skinny and fit is to be prepared. You cannot just walk around here, in the United States, and expect not to be offered junk food items at every turn. Junk food is literally everywhere. Since junk is so easy to get to and so widely available, it is very common for people to just grab junk and mindlessly eat it. This easily obtainable and ready to eat junk is not real food. This junk is not going to satisfy your nutritional needs. Check the label, there is nothing in there. The only thing that this junk does is to momentarily fill your belly while changing your food preferences from natural to unnatural with chemically induced hyper flavors and soft, easy to chew textures that hit every button in your primitive brain causing the dopamine to be dumped in your brain, literally creating and or fueling a junk food addiction and blunting your appetite for real, whole and healthy food that your body actually needs to be healthy.

Junk food has been designed in a laboratory by scientists to literally press all of the happiness buttons in your brain, covering your need for sugar, fat and salt, but missing all of your real nutritional needs. Our bodies are just not sophisticated enough to distinguish between junk and real food until digestion takes place. Then the deficits are noted. The body then notes that real nutrition is missing and sends signals to the brain that even more food is needed because no actual nutrients were obtained with the last load.

Because of the junk that is widely available everywhere we go, it is very important that you eat well and quite a lot of real food before you go anywhere so that you will not be hungry when you arrive at your destination. If you are like me and literally cannot pre-plan, that is okay. Just remember to carry bananas or clementine oranges with you at all times. Have a plan and know where there are some safe fast food choices that you will go to in a hurry if necessary. One of my safe choices is Chipotle's where I get the salad bowl with lettuce, corn, both kinds of beans, salsa, and brown rice. Another fairly safe choice is the Tropical Smoothie Café. Ask for the Caesar wrap with minimal dressing, no cheese and no meat. Many places that you go will have one or two safer choices available. You just have to look and see or ask them to put something together for you specifically. You are worth it.

You have to really think about your goals and what you want your body to look like in a few months. If you keep eating junk food and garbage, you will look like you keep eating junk food and garbage. Real, healthy food will make you look and feel really healthy. Junk food will have less than ten percent of the daily nutrients for any item that is required by the body. When you read the label, it will be clear that this is not real food, just junk. There will be fewer than 10 percent of the daily requirements met for Vitamin C, Vitamin A, Calcium and Iron. Junk food items will have minimal to no fiber and very minimal protein. A good rule of thumb is to not buy anything that is packaged that doesn't supply more than ten percent of your daily nutrient needs for at least two items and make sure that it has less than twenty percent of its calorie content from fat. (Just take the amount of fat grams in the item, multiply this number by ten and then divide this number by the number of total calories in the item. For example, if each serving contains 240 calories and there are 8 fat grams per serving, you take the number of fat grams (8) and multiply this by 10 (rounding up from 9 calories per gram for fat) which gives you 80. You then divide 80 by 240, the total number of calories, and this gives you 0.333, which you then multiply by 100 to get 33.3% of the calories are from fat, so this is an item you pass up as it has more than twenty percent of its calories from fat.

If the item is high in protein or fiber, that makes up for being low in vitamins as long as there is minimal fat (less than 20 percent of the calories come from fat) and it does not have any saturated fat. Nut butters and nuts and seeds in general will be exceptions to this rule as they are often higher in fat. A good rule of thumb is to just avoid packaged items that have labels unless you are in a desperate situation. Sometimes you have to do what you can with what you have and prepare better the next time. Don't beat yourself up over these times but don't let them occur repeatedly either.

Now unless you live alone, this plan can become complicated. The other members of your family will usually not be very happy about this change. They will act like it is great that you want to change and they will pretend to be supportive until you go to the store and they are with you. Theoretically they will be in your corner because who would actually be against someone trying to be healthy? But people can be awfully funny when it comes to their food and junk food is highly addictive. They don't necessarily have to make the change with you but it will certainly be much better if they do. If they are children and you are an adult, then there will be no problem, you are in charge and are the leader and they will have no choice but to do as you tell them as you are the one who calls the shots and pays the bills. Seriously, you are the grown up so act like one and don't be scared of your children. This is much better for them and you know it. They will not die; in fact they will be just fine and even better for not eating junk all day every day.

If you are married and or living with a significant other and this person or your spouse does not agree to do this, it can become really difficult. Sometimes, you can set up shelves and cupboards where they will keep their junk but just knowing the junk is there can make this plan difficult. I have actually had several arguments in the grocery store with my husband when we first began implementing this change. I am sure that we are on video cameras yanking potato chip bags and bakery products back and forth between us. I can't tell you how many times I have removed items from the grocery cart that are not allowed only to find them back on the belt at checkout time, where I removed them again. Remember that you must NOT put anything in the grocery cart that is not allowed. And you must not allow anyone else to do so either, whatever it takes. Don't break down under the whining of the kids and don't give in to the grumbling spouse. Be strong. You are RIGHT! Health is important and must be earned. The only way to do it is to DO IT!

And please don't feel sorry for your family. You are making them healthier and stronger, not depriving them of needed items. They don't need that stuff anymore than you do! It's just as bad for them as it is for you and even if they are not overweight, junk is junk and doesn't help anyone ever. Even skinny people need to eat nutritious food. Even skinny people have clogged arteries and heart attacks. Being skinny or naturally thin doesn't mean that you get to eat junk. Everyone will stay healthier if they eat properly and eating properly always leads to better health for everyone. No one has ever regretted eating right.

When my husband and I first started eating healthier, I let him go into the grocery store by himself one day as I waited in the car with our little poodle, so she wouldn't have to wait alone. When he came out of the store he started loading the bags of groceries into the car and I saw a bag of corn chips in one of the bags. I asked him about the chips and he said that when we had gone out for dinner a few weeks earlier, we had ordered some chips and salsa as an appetizer and since he knew we had salsa at home he thought he would just bring home some chips so we could enjoy them with the salsa. I didn't know what to do. I felt a little panicky as I know the rules are very clear. This was a clear violation of the rule "Do not bring home anything from the grocery store that you are not supposed to eat."

I looked at him and said that he needed to return the chips. He looked confused and then said something about leaving them for the kids to eat. I knew that if those chips came into the house that they would be consumed by my husband and me and that by coming in to the house "just this once' this would lead absolutely nowhere positive. I thought about all of our hard work and all of the positive changes we had made. I couldn't stand to see this start to fall apart right there in the grocery store parking lot, so I grabbed the bag of corn chips and threw it across the parking lot of the store as hard as I could.

I didn't throw the bag because I was angry. I didn't throw the bag because I was upset. I threw the bag to protect both of us from a serious addiction that causes severe health problems. I threw it like one throws a live hand grenade in the opposite direction of their loved ones. I threw it to keep both of us safe in a world that makes it way too easy to indulge in all of the wrong things all of the time. I threw it for the sake of keeping us on the right track, a way of recommitting to the cause. I threw it far away. I hope the seagulls enjoyed their special treat.

When you are in the grocery store, you are going to shop in the perimeter of the store for the most part. You are going to buy any vegetable that you like to eat. You are going to buy any fruit that you like to eat. If you like to cook, you will make homemade beans. If you are like me, canned beans will do. If you like to cook and have time to do so, your options are limitless. If you are on a tight schedule and / or are a lazy cook like me, then your options will be more limited, however it is still quite possible to eat well and be full with a very busy schedule and minimal time. "I don't have time" is not an excuse that I will believe. As long as convenience stores sell bananas, there is no reason to eat junk at fat, I mean fast food restaurants.

Keep in mind, while shopping at grocery stores, that this is where you will win the battle. The grocery store has been designed and especially laid out to entice a consumer into purchasing excessive items, most of which aren't really food at all.

The grocery store or Supermarket as we know it today did not exist until the 1920's. Between 1920 and 1950 Supermarkets began selling processed foods and by the 1950's became the stores that they are today. Supermarket advertisers spend millions of dollars on psychological testing to learn how human beings function and what drives them to make choices to purchase the items that they purchase. Supermarkets contain very few real food items and are mostly conglomerations of overly processed, packaged "food like" substances. It is the goal of the supermarket to entice the consumer, which is you, to buy excessive amounts of processed junk foods made up mostly of fat, sugar and salt with a few other cheap ingredients. This is to maximize the amount of profit that can be made on each food item by the food processing and manufacturing companies. What is good for American companies is not what is good for your health. If you allow food manufacturers, who are only out to make money, choose what food that you and your family eat on a regular basis, you can be sure it will not be what is the healthiest for your bodies.

Because we, as a country, have allowed the food manufacturers to "free" us from the chore of cooking and preparing food over the last thirty years, most people don't even know what real food is anymore. Their entire diet consists of packaged products that they heat and/or add water to at home to manufacture meals made mostly of cheap, white, highly processed starches, fats and sugars placed together in differing quantities with chemical additives used for flavorings and preservatives. People have become so used to this high sugar, highly processed food items that they feel that they cannot survive without them. What is life if one has not tasted and purchased a boxed meal in which one is to add hamburger, tuna or chicken for its completion? What will be for dinner if it isn't a frozen entrée or takeout pizza?

Americans eat more pizza than they eat of almost any other kind of food item. What used to be considered a treat is now considered a staple food, eaten at least a few times per week for both lunch and supper. When people are in a hurry, they grab a pizza. If the kids have after school activities, grab a pizza. If work was really tough today, grab a pizza.

If we all start eating what we should eat instead of what is most profitable for the food manufacturing companies, the large food manufacturers will not be happy about this change. These companies make a lot of money by producing packages in the grocery store that people now consider to be food. The substances inside of these packages contain cheap ingredients that are dressed to look like real food. People buy them, believing that they are feeding their families nutritious meals, but there is nothing nutritious about any kind of packaged macaroni and cheese with canned green beans. If you eat a steady diet of the manufactures "food like substances" there is no way that you will not be depleted of micronutrients and craving more junk. You will think you are eating real food when you are not and you will have toxic hunger and a response to this food that makes you think you need more of it when in fact you don't need it at all and should never eat it again.

Even now there is some pushback by food manufacturing companies and health care professionals to try and diagnose people who refuse to eat junk food with a psychiatric disorder called orthorexia nervosa. This is a ridiculous attempt to make eating healthfully into an illness that requires medication and treatment. Never underestimate the power of eating well to cause others to notice and become alarmed. For some reason when you stop eating junk food and garbage, other people are deeply affected by it and will go to unbelievable lengths to try and pull you back into the fold, even attempting to diagnose you with a ridiculous illness because you won't eat with them at the local greasy fat, I mean fast food burger joint.

The truth is that eating real food is satisfying and delicious in a way that eating processed junk food is not.

You sometimes can take your favorite dish; substitute everything in it for healthier items and still like it! The dish will not taste exactly the same but it will be a version of your favorite and after you have eaten it several times you will like it even more than your old favorite, and more importantly the dish will now be working to improve your health instead of place your health in jeopardy. I have done this for my mom's pancake recipe and for some muffin and other recipes, which you can find in the last chapter of this book. There are many excellent cooks and chefs that are way better than I am at creating healthy versions of not so healthy popular favorite recipes. Two such valuable resources that are easily and readily available for free online are The Brand New Vegan and PotatoStrong. There are, or course, many others, but these two stand out for being free, healthy and easy and for making recipes that are more like the food that most people are used to eating.

When you first change your diet, you will work hard just trying to find things that can become your new favorites. Many times these substitutions will turn out great. Sometimes, though, substitutions will not work. This is why it is impossible to eat most of the desserts in most low fat vegetarian cook books. They are just awful tasting compared to the desserts they are meant to replace. It is best to just understand that these desserts, the ones that were your favorites, are meant for special occasions only, and that special occasions take place about once every two months or so, and certainly not every week.

Saving these very special desserts and food items for truly special occasions works well for some people. Other people find that they have to commit completely to eating healthfully at all times and never look back. You will have to be very honest with yourself about the type of person that you are. With that being said, I don't think that there is anything that tastes better than a piece of ripe, in season fruit. It is nutritious, delicious and satisfies your sweet tooth like nothing else can. If you ever find yourself in a place where cravings for sweets and junk are overwhelming you, eating a large amount of fresh, sweet, whole fruits will usually snap you out of it and satisfy you like nothing else can. For example, eating three bananas and two oranges when you crave a bakery item will usually stop the craving.

So let's take a trip through your average grocery store.

When you first step in the door you are usually greeted with the produce section. This is where the majority of your food purchases will be made. Make sure you pick up carrots, onions, celery, garlic (bottled or fresh, your choice). Usually you can find some bottled prepared ginger next to the bottled garlic. If you like authentic stir fry or Asian inspired dishes pick some of that up too. Pick up some bananas, apples, oranges and potatoes, both sweet and white. Get some broccoli, cabbage, Brussels sprouts, spinach and kale. Purchase mushrooms and bell peppers. Look around and purchase anything that looks interesting to try and that you know you can actually consume in one week.

Don't overbuy. Produce is expensive. Buy enough for the week, remembering that you will have to eat all that you buy within a week or so. Don't under buy; remember this is what you eat all day every day for the most part. Buy organic vegetables if you can, but don't sweat too much if you cannot. Just do the best that you can.

The next section you usually come to contains the nuts and seeds. Make sure you purchase some chia seeds and / or some ground flax seeds to use as egg replacers in baked products. You will need to store the ground flax seed meal in the refrigerator. Purchase some nuts, like walnuts, pecans, sunflower seeds, pistachio nuts, etc. Choose your favorites, keeping in mind that you will eat about one handful a day. The healthiest nuts are raw and unsalted. Be aware that for some reason food manufacturers like to put oil in the nuts that are already oily. Check the labels and avoid these products. If you are currently overweight and trying to slim down it is important to limit your nut portions to a handful a day and no more. If you are very athletic and already thin, you can eat more of them. If you have been eating healthfully for a long time and have not been able to slim down, check the amount of nuts and seeds that you are eating as they are usually responsible for keeping you heavy. Just think about what the squirrels look like right before they hibernate for the winter. They are chubby from eating acorns. You will also be chubby if you eat a lot of nuts and seeds. You will be healthier than other people eating chips and junk, but eating too many nuts and seeds can cause you to remain overweight even when you are eating properly.

When you buy peanut butter, buy only freshly ground peanut butter. This is also true for other nut butters, such as almond and sunflower. I, personally, have a sugar weakness, so I buy the honey roasted, freshly ground peanut butter. Regular peanut butter on the shelf of the average grocery store contains chemicals that keep it from separating at room temperature. These chemicals, like palm oil, are very bad for you and for the environment. The freshly ground peanut butter will stay in peanut butter form for a few weeks at room temperature before it starts to separate. Buy enough that will last for a few weeks, not a few months.

If you like, you can buy low sugar fruit jams or preserves so that you can quickly make a peanut butter and jelly sandwich, but it is really easy (like less than twenty minutes easy) to make your own freezer jam with a fruit pectin product called Sure Jell or Certo, fresh or frozen fruit and sugar. If you are planning to make this, make sure you buy enough fresh or frozen fruit to do so, appropriate containers and of course the Sure Jell or Certo and some sugar. The low sugar or reduced sugar recipe should be followed to try and limit the amount of processed sugar you are eating.

The next section of the grocery store is usually the bakery section. Make sure you buy whole wheat bread, rolls or other bakery goods. You have to make sure that they are made of one hundred percent whole wheat. The label should read, whole wheat, not wheat flour. Wheat flour is just another name for white flour. Whole wheat should be the only flour listed. Read the label. Don't believe the words written on the front of the bakery product or any packaged product for that matter. The labeling on the front is all about marketing and advertising and has little to do with the actual product. Read the nutritional facts label on the back of the product to get the whole truth about what is really in the bread.

The next section you usually come across will be the meat and the deli. Skip all of this. You don't need any meat, cold cuts, cheese or any of the junk food available in this section. Just walk right on through; there is no need to stop. The only thing in this section may be a "Tofurkey" brand sausage, which is a meat analog product you can use as a flavoring agent if you have been a heavy meat eater and are in the process of making the switch. This product and others like it can help you break old habits and you can buy it if you think that you will eat it. Most of the plant based medical practitioners frown on this and it is not to be considered a health food but it may be a necessary "crutch" to get you through the transition. You can also buy tofu if you would like to try it. The silken kind works well for dips, desserts and dressings. The firm one is best for stir fries. I, personally, am not a big tofu eater but my husband loves the stuff.

Canned and dried soups are often so full of sodium that you should never purchase them. Any item that you buy will have an ingredient label and that is where you can learn the truth about what is in there. Names that sounds like chemicals, are chemicals, so don't buy them. It is very simple and easy to make soup at home. It will take you less than twenty minutes from start to finish, especially if you chop up the vegetables with a food processor, so there is really no reason to buy ready-made soups. You can make a big batch of vegetable soup at home, freeze it into one and two cup containers, and easily take it to work or on the go without any difficulty at all. It is a good idea to buy some vegetable broth. Look for the low sodium variety. It is possible to make your own very delicious and nutritious vegetable broth at home which is likely well worth the effort, but for the sake of this plan, we are trying to keep things as easy as possible, so a low sodium variety will work.

The next section you will come to will be the beverages. If you have to drink coffee and you know that you can limit your coffee to one cup a day, then feel free to buy coffee. If you are a coffee addict and cannot limit your intake to one cup a day, then do not buy coffee. Caffeine is not good for you, especially in large quantities. I don't care what the USDA guidelines are on this subject. If it can give you a headache and cause you to have polycystic or lumpy breasts, increase menopausal symptoms and cause addiction then it cannot possibly be a healthy food choice. You can buy tea, regular and green tea, fruit teas, and herbal teas. Feel free to buy any tea that you like and that you think that you will drink.

Do not buy any hot cocoa mixes or fruit juices; do not buy any junk food drinks. You can buy bottled water if that is something that you like to have around. Buy plain bottled water, not energy drinks or artificially flavored waters. If you need the water to be flavored, then squeeze a real lemon or orange in to it. You do not need to buy any nutritional beverages of any kind, like Ensure or Slim Fast or any protein drinks or powders at all. They are not healthful and they are not necessary and in my opinion, are all junk food.

You are going to eat your food and not drink it. You are going to try and drink six to eight glasses of water a day while on this plan. Your food will be less salty than it has been and your food will have higher water content to it but you will still do better if you get enough water to drink throughout the day to keep you well hydrated. You will know that you are well hydrated when you urinate five to six times a day and the urine is light yellow in color.

The next aisle will usually contain the cookies, chips and all types of snacking junk foods. Skip that aisle. All of the crackers you can purchase, with the exception of Engine 2 products, are just a whole lot of processed junk with added oil and chemicals. These items have minimal to no nutritional value. Don't even tempt yourself with this junk. You don't need pretzels; you are going to eat carrot sticks instead. Don't be fooled by items labeled "veggie chips" and items that say they are "baked" for lower fat content. The truth is that all of these are simply junk food that will make you fat, sick and very thirsty. Leave all of this junk at the store. Don't be fooled into buying nutrition bars and all kinds of junk foods that are aimed at people trying to get healthy on the run. Junk food manufacturers pay attention to trends and they will surely try to mask their junk food in ways that make it seem healthy. Don't be fooled, it is all junk food.

The real healthy energy bar is apples, oranges and bananas. That is the real healthy food you can eat while on the run. What you need to eat is an apple or an orange, not a nutritional junk food bar. Nutritional bars are not food, they are junk. If an item contains added oil, it is junk. If an item contains more than a few easily identifiable ingredients, it is junk. Stay away from all junk and do not, under any circumstances, put it in your grocery cart. This is not food. It is junk.

In the snack food aisle there will also be some popcorn. Not microwave popcorn, regular popcorn in a jar. Air popped popcorn is a terrific snack for this eating plan. You can eat as much air popped corn as you like. I often sprinkle mine with "no cheese" sprinkle, salt and pepper. (See the recipe section). All you need is an air popper and you will have a delicious, filling, crunchy snack in just a few minutes. It takes just about the same amount of time to air pop popcorn as it does for the microwave to pop the popcorn that is full of all kinds of chemicals and garbage. Regular brands of microwave popcorn are never an acceptable treat. That is not food. It is chemically laden garbage. Don't eat garbage. There are some brands of microwave popcorn that contain only the popcorn and nothing else. Read the label and you will know.

The next aisle will be the baking aisle. If you like to bake, buy regular or pastry whole wheat flour or white whole wheat flour. Make sure the label says whole wheat, not just wheat flour. Buy some envelopes of quick rising yeast so you can make your own no fat added pizza crust. Buy stone ground cornmeal if you like cornbread or muffins, baking soda, baking powder, salt, pepper, sugar and any spices that you think you will need. Spices like onion powder, chili powder, garlic powder, Mrs. Dash, in all of her many varieties, dried basil, dried oregano, Italian Seasoning,

Herbs de Provence, dried dill, ginger, cinnamon, cumin, turmeric, curry powder, rosemary, thyme, parsley and sage. Herbs and spices are what you will use to really make your food come to life. After eating healthfully for some time I now know why the spice trade was so important in previous centuries. I now know why men would travel hundreds and thousands of miles, risking everything, including their lives, to obtain the spices that we can now get just by going to our nearest grocery store. Spices absolutely make a world of difference between a bland and boring barely edible dish and a food that you savor and look forward to eating again. Don't be shy with the use of your spices; they will really make your new foods delicious.

Another thing you will need in the baking aisle is nutritional yeast. It is gold in color. If you cannot find it at your usual grocery store, look around or order in online. Nutritional yeast is really good to have on hand as it lends a "cheesy" and "buttery" flavor to many dishes. As a group of healthy eating people, we really have to come up with a better name for it as nutritional yeast does not sound very appetizing or tasty, but trust me; it tastes much better than it sounds.

Do not buy any cake or brownie mixes, muffin mixes or any other junk that crowds this aisle. Do not buy sugar substitutes. Regular table sugar contains fifteen calories in a teaspoon and fifty calories in a tablespoon. You are not going to be eating so much sugar that this will make you fat.

Sugar and salt are okay on this eating plan in very small, controlled quantities. Sugar and salt can make food taste better. You will try to decrease the amount that you need, but if you like it, use real sugar and not sugar substitutes. Sugar substitutes are just a disgusting chemical junk food that even the ants won't touch. They know it is bad for them, shouldn't we know as well?

While you are in the baking aisle pick up some canned pumpkin and unsweetened apple sauce that you can use as oil substitutes that baked good recipes often call for. Do not buy any oil. Not olive oil, not canola oil, not safflower oil, not coconut oil. You do not need any oil. Oil is junk food. Buy some parchment paper so you can make baked goods that do not stick to the pans despite their lack of oil, but do not buy oil.

In the ethnic foods section you will want to buy dried beans if you have time to cook them or if you are on a seriously tight budget as they are very inexpensive. In any case, all different colors of lentils cook very fast and you should have them on hand for quick soups and stews. Brown rice is also a kitchen staple to have on hand if you like to eat it. Traditional brown rice takes one hour to cook and it is best cooked in a rice cooker. Don't buy white rice for the same reason that you don't buy white flour. All of the nutrients and fiber have been stripped away in the refining process and you are basically buying junk. You can also find mixed grain rice and wild rice which are both also really delicious and nutritious. I go to an Asian grocery store and buy brown Jasmine rice as it is especially fragrant during the cooking process and is very tasty and delicious. In the last few months I have found a new kind of brown rice that cooks in thirty minutes instead of sixty which really helps on busy weeknights. The nutritional value in the quick cooking brown rice is supposed to be equivalent to the regular brown rice. The flavor is not quite as good but it is a good variety to have on hand if you need to eat in a hurry. Do not buy any of the boxed rice products, like Ricearoni, Uncle Bens, or any of the Lipton quick cooking varieties. Do not buy any packaged dinners, like Hamburger and Tuna Helper or Macaroni and Cheese. These are all highly processed, packaged junk foods with no nutritional value and have no place in a healthy diet.

The ethnic grocery store aisle will also have refried beans, corn tortillas with minimal fat and whole grain, low fat tortilla wraps if you like eating wraps instead of sandwiches. Hopefully you can find the vegetarian low fat refried beans. If you cannot find them, then opt for the low fat refried beans over the vegetarian beans as having low fat is more important than being strictly vegetarian. Also this is the aisle that will have the low sodium tamari sauce or low sodium soy sauce. These are really good to have on hand for flavoring quick stir fry dishes.

The next aisle will be the condiments and salad toppings. Do not buy any oils or mayonnaise. Do not buy "vegan" mayonnaise. It is still full of fat and oil. No refined oil is good for you. Olive oil is not a health food despite what you may have heard. A "serving" of oil is usually 2 tablespoons. Two tablespoons of oil contained 240 calories. 240 calories! That's crazy! and all of it is FAT! Oil has absolutely no nutritional value and does not contribute to your health in any way. I would rather waste 240 calories on a Snickers Bar instead of 2 tablespoons of oil. You would be better off eating a Snickers bar than you would be eating oil. Oil is just extra calories and has no nutritional value. You do not need any added oil in your diet, no matter what you have been told, and it is seriously just junk food. This means no coconut oil and no olive oil. This means not even extra virgin cold pressed olive oil. It is all bad.

People always think that they need some fat in their diet or they will die. The truth is that all foods contain small amounts of fat put together by nature in their most perfect and easily digestible form. Bananas have fat, carrots have fat; all foods contain some amount of fat, even lettuce. You do not need to add extra fat to your diet. If you are eating real food, you will get exactly as much fat as your body needs and no more. Fat, in the form of oil, contains 4000 calories per pound. Even a small drizzle of it will add an incredible amount of extra calories to your food. One tablespoon of oil contains 120 calories. That is 120 extra calories that nobody needs. The average person eats between 400 and 700 extra calories per day just from oil added to their food.

People are very addicted to oil and added fats in general and this can be a really hard step for some people, but remember that there is no need to add extra fat to anything that you cook. It will take about eight to ten weeks of healthful eating for you to lose your craving for excessive fat, but eventually this craving will go away. At first it feels like something is missing, but you will get used to this. In fact, later, when someone feeds you something at a party or you eat at a restaurant, you will easily be able to tell that there is added oil in a dish. In this food plan, we will get our fat calories from whole foods, and not from highly refined oil products.

People often think that they need to use oil to cook their food in pans. The food will not stick to your pans while you stir fry it if you heat the pan well before adding the food to it and then moisten the pan with vegetable broth, water, beer, wine, vinegar or any other liquid you can think of. To obtain the most flavor during cooking, I first dry sauté the onions and garlic until lightly browned in a hot pan and then I use the vegetable broth, water, beer, wine, vinegar or any other liquid you can think of as I add the other ingredients to keep the other ingredients from sticking. I do use non-stick pans to cook my food. Parchment paper can be used in baking pans to keep food from sticking to the inside. I use a ceramic waffle iron that

196

works well to keep the waffle from sticking to the waffle iron.

When switching to a very healthy diet it may at first be necessary to use a commercially available salad dressing to help you get used to eating salads on a regular basis. Salad dressings are really manufactured junk food products and should be used with extreme caution. If you absolutely cannot eat salad without dressing, then choose a no fat dressing and serve it on the side, dipping only your fork tines into it instead of pouring the dressing on top of the salad. It is very easy to make salad dressing at home using freshly squeezed fruit juices, spices and all kinds of vinegars that will be much better for you than any commercially available dressing.

You can buy sliced black olives in this aisle too if you like them, for taco salads. If you like flavored vinegars, this is where you can find them. Experiment with different kinds of vinegars to find your favorites. This aisle also has pickles. Use them sparingly, as flavoring agents. They aren't a health food, but they aren't terrible either. The same goes for ketchup and barbecue sauce. Buy the kind of ketchup and barbecue sauce that does not contain high fructose corn syrup. Mustard of any kind is also fine. While you are in the condiment aisle, if you like to eat pancakes and waffles, buy some real maple syrup. Get the kind that really comes out of a tree. It is very expensive but you are not buying any meat anymore and this will be well worth it.

The next aisle will be the cans and pastas. Do not buy canned vegetables. They are worthless garbage and contain no nutritional value whatsoever. They don't even have any fiber and contain quite a lot of sodium. Canned vegetables are worse than useless. You can buy canned beans, black beans, canellini beans, kidney beans, black eyed peas, garbanzo beans, etc. Try to get the low sodium varieties. You can also make these fresh using dried beans, which are much less expensive, but if, like me, you are a lazy cook or are short on time then canned beans can really help out and are good to have around. Manufacturers have been responding to peoples fear of BPA in canned foods and you can now find boxes of beans instead of cans. Boxes are better than cans, for health reasons, so if they are available, buy them instead. Before you use canned beans in any recipe, you should place them in a strainer and rinse them off under water to remove most of the salt that is added during the canning process. For that reason you shouldn't bother buying the flavored canned beans, just the regular ones will do. You can also buy canned, or boxed, low salt tomato products. Canned low salt diced tomatoes, canned tomato sauce and canned tomato paste are all really good staples to have on hand for making pasta sauces, soups, chili, and pizza. Again, try to find the low sodium varieties and buy the organic low sodium varieties if your budget allows.

Buy only one hundred percent whole wheat pasta. If you like to eat pasta, and who doesn't, get rotini, spaghetti and lasagna noodles all containing one hundred percent whole wheat. If you have Celiac disease, like two percent of the population does, then you will have to buy and use only gluten free products. There is an additional four to five percent of the populations that is gluten sensitive but not allergic. The rest of us do not need to avoid gluten. If you would like to avoid gluten, it will certainly be much easier to do so now than it ever has been before due to the unnecessary current gluten hysteria that is going on, but understand that most people will not have any trouble digesting gluten. So unless you are one of the two to seven percent of people in the population that have been diagnosed with Celiac disease or have gluten intolerance, feel free to eat whole wheat pasta. It is delicious, comforting, filling and makes eating healthfully a whole lot easier. If you are worried about the impact of GMO's on your health, then buy organic whole wheat pasta products. Organic products, by definition, cannot contain GMO's.

The next aisle will be the cereal products. Buy some oatmeal, steel cut if you like it and have time to cook it, otherwise regular old fashioned oats will do. Don't buy quick cooking oats or instant oatmeal with added sugar. Making oat meal or other hot cereal in the morning takes less than five minutes. You have time to do this. You don't need to buy the quick cooking products in the envelopes that you just add water to. The regular cooking cereals take five minutes or less. The quick cooking products will save you exactly four minutes. If you are cutting the time that close, perhaps a couple of bananas and some whole wheat toast will work better as a breakfast for you.

Buy some yellow whole grain grits, if you like grits as a cereal for breakfast. Yellow corn grits are also useful for making a cheese like topping for pizza and lasagna so they are good to have on hand. You can also buy brown rice cereal, mixed whole grain hot cereals, or any other whole grain hot cereal mix that is available if you like to eat hot cereal for breakfast. You can buy muesli if you like cold cereal. Most of the granolas that are available contain an enormous amount of added fat so make sure that you read the label, checking for added oils and fats. Cereal should be made of whole grains only and not contain any added sugar or added fats and / or oils. Most of the cereals in the cereal aisle will be off limits. Do not be fooled by the packaging, read the nutrition label and see what is really in the cereal box before you buy it.

Next you will run into the dairy section that also usually contains the fresh juices and eggs. You are not going to buy any juice. The reason is that it is not real juice. The orange juice that you buy at the grocery store is made in this way. First, the fresh oranges are picked off of the tress and then they are squeezed and their juice is obtained. At that moment, you have fresh juice. If you can buy it this fresh, then you can buy some juice. Just be careful not to drink too much of it as it is very high in calories but is also very nutritious. If you cannot find genuinely just made today fresh squeezed and pressed juices, then do not bother to buy them at all. You see when the fruit is picked and then pressed or squeezed, you have fresh, healthy juice. Then the manufacturer takes that fresh juice and boils it, also known as pasteurization, and then stores it in large vats after removing all of the oxygen from it for four to six months at a time. When it is time for the juice to be used it is re-oxygenated and colored using orange peels and then a "flavoring packet" is added to make the ugly gray liquid taste and look like fresh squeezed orange juice once again. Sounds delicious, doesn't it? The only way that you can obtain real healthy fruit juice is to buy the real fruit and squeeze it yourself at home. However, drinking juice will only make you fat, as the juice does not contain the fiber found in the whole fruit. I am not sure about the process for making apple juice but the truth is that you need to eat the entire apple. If you are going to use apple, grape or other fruit juices, do so very sparingly, as favoring agents for nutritious whole fruits and vegetables and avoid drinking just the juice as the fiber and other nutrients that belong to the whole fruit are missing. So for the purpose of this eating plan you will only use small amounts of real fresh juice that you have squeezed yourself at home as flavoring agents for salads or in other recipes as needed. You should buy a small hand held citrus juicer to use for this purpose.

You will not be buying any eggs or dairy products. You will not be buying any butter, margarine or other butter substitutes, not even "vegan butter". After reading the book, "The China Study", written by Dr. T. Colin Campbell and his son, Dr. Thomas Campbell, there is no way I can ever recommend that anybody eat dairy products ever again. After I read this book I literally opened my refrigerator and threw away the milk, butter and cheese that were in it. Since then I have eaten very small amounts of dairy products outside of my home on very rare occasions, but there is no way I can regularly feed dairy products to myself or my family with a clear conscience. The scientific evidence on this cannot be clearer.

You can buy some plant based milk. Plant based milks, like almond, cashew and soy milk do not contain any dairy products. The market on plant based milks has really opened up and so many different kinds are now available so it will just be a matter of experimentation for you to find out which ones you like the best. Try to choose plant milks that are relatively low in fat and calories and choose ones that are fortified with Vitamin D. Always read the label. For instance coconut milk contains saturated fat that you may not want to ingest, especially if you have any type of heart disease or high cholesterol. I, personally, really like light soy milk for baking and cooking and unsweetened almond / coconut milk or cashew milk for my breakfast cereal. I also really like to drink an occasional glass of chocolate flavored almond milk as a treat and chocolate flavored almond milk can also be placed in an ice cream maker and comes out with a consistency and taste that is very similar to a Wendy's chocolate frosty when it is finished. This is a really delicious treat. You can also make coconut ice cream with full fat coconut milk but this is for only very special occasions as it is full of fat.

The next section of the grocery store will be the freezer cases. You can buy frozen vegetables if you did not find the ones you liked in the fresh produce section. There are many varieties of frozen vegetables that are so easy to cook. You just pop them in the microwave for a few minutes in the bag they came in and they are ready to eat. If you get home late and don't have time to make a real supper, these microwaved bags of vegetables work well. Simply steam them, top them with "no cheese" sprinkle (see recipe section) and serve them alongside some leftover mashed potatoes or already cooked brown rice or other whole grains.

The freezer section of the store will also contain already made veggie burgers and other meat analog products, like veggie sausage patties, barbecued veggie riblets, veggie "bacon" strips and soy protein "crumbles" made to resemble hamburger. When you are first starting out on your journey to eating a healthy plant based diet, these foods may have their place but cannot be considered true health foods. They can be especially useful if you are having trouble with reluctant family members. Using these meat analog products can help you to navigate more successfully into the world of plant based food living and eating. I would not suggest that you eat these products daily; once or twice a month should be sufficient. They should be eaten in very small quantities and used mostly as flavoring agents for the actually nutritious vegetables and grains. Do not buy any ice cream or frozen desserts of any kind. Fresh fruit will be your dessert for now.

There. You made it through the grocery store and you are now ready to make meals that are fast, easy and delicious and will make you skinny and fit and glowing with health.

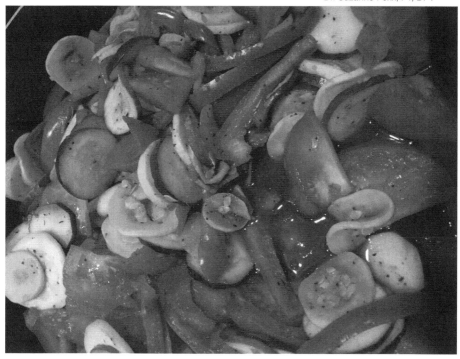

Chapter 6: Putting The Plan Into Action:

How To Be Skinny And Fit And What It Looks Like On A Daily Basis

Alright, you made it through and have decided to implement a healthy eating plan and make it into a real plan that you and your family can live with, and I do mean really live with. You are going to try this for six weeks and have made up your mind to do it. With new information you have changed your attitude. You now know the difference between real food and junk food. You now fully understand that the reason we eat is to nourish our bodies and not to make them sick and you have decided that ninety seven percent of the time or more that you will eat only real foods that makes you healthy and not junk foods that makes you sick.

You have picked through the grocery store and have purchased some staples and you are ready to really get going. You know why you are doing this and you are now ready to really get started. So where are you mentally? Do you really want to change or are you still at the "thinking it through" stage. Change is change and by its very nature it will be difficult but it isn't really that hard once you are mentally ready to do it.

Keep in mind that this plan isn't difficult when you have set yourself up to mentally do it. It will be fairly straight forward and easy to do once you have changed your mind about what is and what isn't food. Food is meant to nourish your body and make you healthy, not to make you sick and fat. It really doesn't matter so much what you eat on your birthday, Christmas, Thanksgiving, the Fourth of July, the Memorial Day Picnic, etc. It really matters what you eat the other three hundred and fifty five days of the year. It turns out that changing your mind about what is and isn't food and the proper role of food in your life is the most difficult part of the whole process. Once you realize what food is and start to use it as a tool to heal your body, you can really eat in a healthy way that will make you live a long and healthy life and look amazing while you do it.

The plan that I propose does not require suffering and starvation or unrealistic goals and expectations. It is real. It takes minimal effort but it does require a change in your mental state.

And now, the rules:

First and foremost you must always remember to eat when you are hungry. Do not go hungry. Have a piece of fruit, another salad, carrots or celery sticks, a handful of nuts, or a healthy smoothie, make a meal Eat however much you like of any kind of vegetable, bean, fruit and / or whole grain. I repeat, DO NOT GO HUNGRY. Being hungry is not a part of this plan. Being hungry will set you up for failure. Being hungry will cause you to become irritable and easily give up. Keep in mind that food cravings and addictions are very real and you will likely be suffering from your previous poor choices for the next several weeks as you battle to restore your body to balance and health. You will likely encounter "toxic hunger" for the first three days and then have cravings for fatty junk food items because you, like most others, are actually addicted to junk food. Cravings for fatty, unhealthy foods can last for eight to ten weeks. Being hungry is not part of this plan. Being hungry will not help you attain your goals and you have enough to deal with without being hungry. So do not ever go hungry.

It is also important to keep in mind that if you are following the rules, there won't be any room for poor food choices. If you are following the rules and doing your best to eat all of the things that you are supposed to eat on a daily basis, then there really isn't a whole lot of room for eating garbage. As an example, if you eat a large bowl of oatmeal, covered with plant based milk and two bananas and go to the office and someone brings in doughnuts, your stomach simply will not have room to eat them. If you manage to take one bite, you won't be craving another as you will already be full. In fact you may be able to taste the hydrogenated oil in the doughnuts and it will make you ill and disgusted just thinking about what it is doing to your arteries and after having looked at your gorgeous new body in the mirror while you were getting ready to leave for work, you will simply decide not to eat the doughnuts.

But, if you skipped this rule, rushed out of the house, forgot to eat breakfast and then saw the doughnuts, your natural hunger drive will kick in and of course you will eat the doughnuts. In fact you will probably eat two or more of them. Following these rules can really save you in these types of circumstances. By eating a whole lot of nutritious and healthy foods, you will not have room for the junk food that is literally everywhere.

Here is another situation that may occur. You go to the office and it is somebodies birthday so to celebrate everyone decides to go out to lunch. You want to go with them. At the restaurant everyone is ordering chicken tenders, mashed potatoes and fajitas but you have not eaten your big salad yet today so in order to put a check mark next to this requirement, you order the big salad, no cheese, dressing in a cup on the side and then proceed to eat all of the complimentary pumpernickel bread, without butter of course, while your co—workers stare in amazement that you ate all of the bread but are the size of a bread stick. You then order the spaghetti with marinara sauce as your entrée and proceed to eat the whole plate; again your co-workers don't know what to say. In this case the spaghetti pasta was likely made with white spaghetti and not whole wheat and there is likely some added oil in the marinara sauce, but the important part is that you stuck to the rules as much as was possible under the circumstances and enjoyed a lovely social event with your co-workers. This is not about pushing a vegan agenda or making other people uncomfortable around you. Food and good company are to be enjoyed. It is just much easier to enjoy food that you know is making you healthy instead of contributing to disease and / or making you fat and sick. This is the very best way to have your (whole wheat, no egg, no oil, no dairy) cake and eat it too.

Here are the 9 Rules you can really live with:

<u>Rule 1: Do not ever put anything in your grocery cart that will make you sick instead of making you healthy.</u>

Do not bring any food into the house that is making you sick instead of making you better. Ask yourself, "Is this food? Or is this junk?" If it is junk, do not allow yourself or your family members to bring it into the house as it will be way too easy to slip back into old deeply ingrained eating habits. If you are living with others who are refusing to go along with your eating plan, designate an area for this person to store the junk food (perhaps the locked trunk of their car?) that will not be easily obtainable to you and will be out of your line of sight. Hopefully, by keeping this junk out of your sight it will be out of your mind. This only applies to adults in the house, such as roommate's or spouses. Your children don't count as they do not buy the food and you must be gentle but firm with them serving them and preparing for them the same meals to eat that you are eating yourself. Remember that you are doing this to improve the health of everyone and it is really in their best interest. You are their parent. Your children will be healthier and happier and ultimately they will thank you later when they don't have to deal with acne, heart disease, diabetes and many forms of cancer like their junk food eating peers. If they have a serious dislike of the new food they can always have peanut butter and jelly sandwiches or cereal. Ask them to join you in your new journey but don't force them to eat the food.

Rule 2: Avoid eating all processed food.

Processed junk food is everywhere and this will be the most difficult part of this plan. This step is not easy but it is absolutely essential. If the item you are about to eat is in a package and the ingredient list contains any item that is difficult to read, then this is processed garbage and not real food. If the item you are about to eat contains palm oil, hydrogenated oil, etc., it is processed junk and will only make you sick. If the item you are about to eat is not real food but is manufactured and more than twenty percent of its calories come from fat and it does not contain any fiber, don't eat it. Processed garbage masquerading as food includes health and nutrition bars, fruit snacks, bottled juices, meal replacement shakes and anything else that is MANUFACTURED instead of being made by nature.

Rule 3: Drink water.

You need to drink six to eight glasses per day. Stop drinking soda and juice. Drink water or unsweetened green, hibiscus or other herbal teas if you cannot stand the taste of water. If you absolutely must add sugar to your green or herbal tea in order to drink it then go ahead and add one to two teaspoons (real sugar contains only fifteen calories per teaspoon but does give you "toxic hunger" symptoms after it digests so be prepared to deal with that if you cannot drink your tea without sugar) and keep working hard to decrease the amount of sugar that you need until you can drink it without added sugar or sweetener. Do not use chemical artificial sweeteners as you are trying to get healthy and that is not a good way to do it. Whole books can be written about the dangers of these Frankenfood type items. Juice is not a healthy option, eat your food and don't drink it.

Rule 4: Stop drinking caffeine.

It is really making you tired. It is bad for your heart and is not helpful to your health. If you really, really must, you can have one cup of coffee in the morning with plant based milk as creamer but understand that the caffeine might make your heart race, gives you lumpy breasts, menopausal hot flash symptoms, and or headaches and if it gives you hypertension or raises your cholesterol; you will have to let it go. I don't care what the latest government recommendations say, if a substance is capable of giving you headaches, fatigue, lumpy breasts, increasing menopausal symptoms and hypertension as well as making your heart race and raising your cholesterol, this cannot be a healthy food and it is not a good food choice. Sorry Starbucks. You're making everyone fat, sick and unhealthy.

Rule 5: Eat a large salad every day.

Eat a large salad every day and some steamed or raw cruciferous vegetable serving every day for either lunch or supper. When I say large, I mean LARGE. This salad should be made up of vegetables, any and all kinds that you enjoy eating, and the salad should not contain any cheese or croutons. At first you may need a small amount of salad dressing to make the salad go down, but as you get used to eating a healthier diet, you can cut down and eventually eliminate all of the dressing or make homemade flavorful dressings that are fat fee and better for you. If you have to eat dressing, dip your fork in a small cup of the dressing to obtain the flavor of the dressing without pouring it all over the leaves of the salad. You can put chopped up nuts or seeds, no more than a handful, on top of the salad as well. In fact, you should make it a point to eat a handful of nuts or seeds every day as part of a really healthy diet. But remember, a handful is all you need, unless you are very active and athletic and already very thin. Eating too many nuts and seeds will keep you from getting skinny and fit. After a few weeks of eating a very large salad every day you will feel weird if you have not eaten your salad. You will feel like something is missing.

Rule 6: Eat 4 – 6 pieces of fresh whole fruit every day.

Eat two to three or more pieces of fresh whole fruit for breakfast every morning and another two to three pieces of fruit in the afternoon for a snack or after dinner for dessert. Do not eat dried fruit or drink fruit juice. Eat real, whole pieces of ripe, delicious fruit. You can make it into a smoothie if you like but use the whole, fresh fruit. Remember that you are a very fancy primate and you need to eat several pieces of fruit every day. Fruit contains micronutrients and fiber that are essential for your good health. You will notice after a few months of doing this that you will actually feel like something is missing and you will crave the freshness of the fruit if you don't eat it every day. This is especially true if you have a sweet tooth. The reason you are craving sugar and candy is because your body needs the nutrients that are contained in fresh, whole fruit. If you are craving sugar or sticky sweet bakery products try to eat two to three pieces of fresh, whole, ripe fruit and then see if you still need that piece of candy, cookie, baked product, etc. You will probably find that the craving is gone.

Rule 7: Always eat breakfast.

You have a lot of work to do and it is important that you have the energy to get it done. Eat some oatmeal, eat whole wheat bread with freshly ground peanut butter or low sugar jam, eat vegan pancakes or waffles, or eat cold whole food cereals with soy, almond or coconut milk. Eat a few pieces of fruit. The important part is that you eat breakfast. Always eat breakfast. Everybody has time to peel and eat two bananas while running out the door or driving to work.

Rule 8: Whole Grains Only.

It is okay to eat as many whole grain, no oil added items that you like. Eat lots and lots of potatoes, sweet and white. Say yes to whole wheat pasta, whole wheat pancakes and waffles, brown rice and whole wheat bread and / or rolls. These items are delicious, filling, very comforting and nutritious. Eating whole grains and starches releases the chemical serotonin in your brain that makes you happy. Eat as much of these whole grain products and starches that you need to. These are the good carbs. They are full of fiber, which will make you feel full and they contain B vitamins and other nutrients. In a pinch, white bread and pasta will have to do, like when you are at a restaurant or out with friends, but at home and when you have a choice, make it whole grain, with no added oil, dairy or eggs. Eat real potatoes, not the kind that come from a box.

Rule 9: Exercise.

You will need to exercise three to five hours a week. You can do it five days a week for an hour or three days a week for one and a half hours, or any other combination that has you exercising at least three to five hours per week. It is only three to five hours. This is less than two percent of the hours you have available to you during the week. It is not that hard. I know that you can do it. Just make the commitment and do it. When you look terrific in your swimsuit, be sure to send me a picture. This will do nothing but make you very happy.

If you follow these nine rules ninety five to one hundred percent of the time, each day, every day, you will be amazed by how fast any excess weight drops off, how health problems disappear and how good you look and feel. Weigh yourself a couple of times a week and keep a log as it will be really neat to look back later and see how fast this worked and how easy it was to do once your mind was set up to actually do it.

Here is an example of eating on this plan that is very nutritious, very filling, and good tasting and easy to do.

Breakfast

1 cup of old fashioned oat meal cooked in 1 ½ cups of water for 5 minutes

1/2 cup almond milk

2 teaspoons of brown sugar

3 oranges

1 banana

5 large strawberries

1/2 cup blueberries.

Lunch

1 twelve inch veggie Subway Sandwich on wheat bread, no cheese, vinegar dressing

1-2 bananas

1 orange

Snack

1-2 bananas.

Dinner

Taco Salad 2 large bowls.

Taco salad made from a whole can of vegetarian fat free refried beans

1 head of romaine lettuce

Small can of sliced black olives

Cherry tomatoes

Green onions

Handful of raw unsalted walnuts

There is no way you can eat the above menu and still be hungry. Your stomach will be mechanically full and filled with proper nutrition. That is a lot of food. Everything was delicious and wholesome and full of nutrients.

Here is another day:

Breakfast:

3 oranges

2 bananas

½ cup of yellow corn grits cooked in 1 ½ cups of water for 5 min

2 tsp. of sugar

½ cup of almond /coconut milk

Lunch:

Smoothie from the Tropical Smoothie Café, no sugar or only ½ sugar added

Salad from Tropical Smoothie Café, No cheese, no dressing

Sprinkled with "no cheesy" sprinkle (see recipes)

Supper:

2 large bowls of vegetable chili (see recipes)

Over 1 cup of mixed whole grain rice

Sprinkled with "no cheesy" sprinkle (see recipes)

5 cups of strawberries for dessert

This menu was also was very filling and very satisfying.

Here is another day

Breakfast:

1 cup of Old Fashioned Oatmeal cooked for 5 min in 1 ½ cups water

2 tsp of sugar

½ cup almond / coconut milk

2 bananas

Lunch:

Large Salad from grocery store salad bar

Fork dipped in low fat dressing for each bite of salad

1 small can of Bush's vegetarian baked beans with sprinkle of cinnamon added

1 Apple

Supper:

2 cups of whole grain rice

3 cups of steamed baby carrots and broccoli

Mrs. Dash and a splash of Low sodium tamari sauce

And another day:

Breakfast:

1 cup of quick cooking yellow corn grits

½ cup of coconut / almond milk

2 teaspoons of sugar

5 clementine oranges

Lunch at Chipolte's Mexican Gill

The salad with all the different beans, grilled peppers, brown rice, corn and salsa

Supper

1 ½ cups of brown rice

2 cups of stir sautéed vegetables with sauce topped with peanuts (see recipes)

2 bananas

Can you see this? This is not at all difficult. It is not at all time consuming. It can easily fit into any schedule. If you fail to plan ahead, like I very often do, it is not hard to find items on the go that will work. They are not perfect, but with a few tweaks, they will work.

A question I am often asked is can you eat out healthfully at fat, I mean fast food restaurants? The answer is only if you make your choices very carefully, keeping in mind that most burger joints are just a bad idea especially in the beginning when you are first getting used to new routines. There just isn't anything at McDonalds that is okay except for the large salad but because it isn't very popular, it won't be terribly fresh or delicious. You just will not have the willpower to not fall into your usual routine once you are confronted with the items you used to eat on a regular basis. So for the most part, fat, I mean fast food restaurants, with very few exceptions, are almost always a bad choice. This is because there are almost no healthy options available in them and because there are so many highly palatable forbidden items so easily available to you once you step in the door. So for this reason it is really not a good idea to even enter them or make them a part of your daily plan.

The funny part is that once you have lost your excessive weight you won't even want to go into these types of places because you won't ever want to go back to the way that things were. You will have worked too hard to achieve your goals and that kind of food will taste exactly like what it is...garbage; just empty calories without any real nutritional value. This is food that will make you sick instead of making you well. Mentally, you will have changed, and there is no way you will want to eat those items.

With that being said, fat, I mean fast food is widely available for a reason. Most of us work long hours and don't have a lot of extra time to make food from scratch at home. For that reason, I personally visit Subway, The Tropical Smoothie Café, Jason's Deli and Chipotle's a few times each per week. Most of the items available in these places are also junk food and not very good for you. When going to any restaurant, just use your head and your common sense to choose the most healthful options that are available. Some of the larger grocery stores have really nice salad bars and if you buy and carry small cans of vegetarian baked beans and with the addition of a few pieces of fruit, this can be a very healthy and delicious weekday work day meal.

If you are invited to a social event where you know that there will be food that you simply cannot and do not want to say no to, make sure that you go to the party prepared. You should make it a point to eat a large healthy meal before you arrive at the event you are planning to attend that you know will contain food that is not good for you but will be highly palatable and extremely tempting. For example, I was invited out to eat to a Hibachi Grill type place where the oil covers everything. I ate a large portion of oatmeal and two bananas before going. I ate the first course, the Miso Soup and after that I was pretty full. I picked at my meal, had it boxed up and then "forgot" to take the box home with me. This works well so that you don't attract a lot of unwanted attention in social gatherings. Most people, unless they are very strong willed, cannot stand up to the type of scrutiny that a healthy diet causes. If people notice and ask, just brush it off and ask them about their lives. Dr. Doug Lisle, co-author of the book "The Pleasure Trap" says to tell them that you are just trying something that likely won't work and how did they do on the project they were working on anyway? Just change the subject and keep it light. If you go to a party and have "pre" eaten, you can then taste the treats that will inevitably be available but you won't be stuffing them in your mouth hand over fist because you will simply be too full to eat them. In that way, you can have your cake and eat it too. You will not be hungry enough to eat all kinds of garbage, but eating very small amounts of your absolute favorites on a special occasion is not what caused you to be fat and sick. This kind of indulgence is called being human. If you do it in a very controlled and careful way, it cannot make you fat and sick. If you are the type of person who cannot stop eating these items once you start then you will just have to say no and leave it at that. Another smart idea is to bring one to two carefully prepared dishes with you to the party that you know you will be able to eat and enjoy so that you will not make a spectacle of yourself walking around with your empty plate.

With that being said, it is important that you not let the way that you eat become part of more than the most casual of party conversations. Try not to get into conversations and debates about it while you are attending social functions. Just breezily say, "Well, it seems to be working for me...I'm just trying an experiment..." and quickly change the subject back to a topic relevant to the party or person with whom you are speaking.

It is never a good idea to allow yourself to be cornered and grilled about your weight loss strategies while keeping social company as the inevitable situation will be that the people you are with will always feel judged and will be angry, agitated and irritable with you concerning this diet plan that is so obviously working and working well.

If you wish to keep your social life afloat while eating healthfully, keep your conversations about the way you eat and what you are doing to restore your health to the minimal amount that is possible. If people persist in discussing your weight loss or demand answers, suggest that you make later plans at a different time or place to discuss your transformation at length. People can become very upset when they find out what you are doing and it can seriously put a damper on your social life if you do not go about it quietly and carefully. Most people, especially women, want to please others, and controversial diets can be very uncomfortable, especially if they are noticeably working. As Dr. Doug Lisle says, just keep it light and casual and try to get the attention off of you as quickly as possible. Say things like, "Well it seems to be working for now, I am sure that you don't want to hear about it" and change the subject.

I attended a party recently where I was talking with some of the other guests, two of whom had recently lost large amounts of weight. I was pretty excited to find out how they had done this, as I thought it might have been through this whole foods plan as I had worked with one of their fathers and he had lost sixty pounds in a four month period following the plan in this book. I asked them how they had lost the weight and they said that they used meal replacement shakes followed by a sensible dinner. I asked them why they had not followed the plan that their father had followed and they said that he was on some maniacally crazy, very restrictive diet with an unbelievable amount of exercise and that they didn't feel that this was even a possibility for normal, average people to do. They felt that their father had to have had a tremendous amount of self-control in order to keep up with the plan.

I then let them know that their father had actually followed the plan in this book, which really isn't that restrictive or difficult and that he had performed only three to five hours or exercise a week and that he and I, along with my husband, had lost weight together and, more importantly I think, have all maintained the weight loss. This plan is very easy to implement once you make up your mind about what is and isn't food. However, most people will say, "This kind of eating plan simply can't be done". In fact that leads us to:

Reason number one why people choose not to eat healthfully

I was talking to my very closest friend about this and this is what she had to say about the subject:

"I can't believe that you keep trying to get people to eat the way that you do. You probably don't even have any taste buds anymore because all of that stuff that you recommend that people eat tastes like cardboard! You probably can't even taste that stuff anymore because you have been eating that way for so long. You probably can't even remember what REAL food tastes like. Every time I try to eat something that you say is supposed to be good for you I just gag and I can't eat it. Nobody likes it; none of the kids, not my husband and certainly not me. Nobody wants to eat it. I don't care if it is better for you, I am only going to live on this earth one time and I don't want to feel like I am being tortured every day when all I want to do is get something to eat. As a result of all of your pushing and all of the things you have said I have markedly increased my intake of fruits and vegetables and I eat honey oat wheat bread now instead of white bread. I eat a salad almost every day for lunch and I do feel a little better but if I want to put cheese, meat and salad dressing on my salad and eat cheese, milk, meat, white bread and processed foods every day then so be it. I am going to and I don't want to hear you talk about how bad it is for me. My kids and I have a lot to do and they have to eat something before they go to their activities. They don't want to eat fruit and they don't like the food and I just don't have the energy to fight with them constantly. I do eat a mostly healthy diet and I am sick of hearing you criticize everything I eat, like I am constantly making bad choices. This is how everyone in America eats and that is just the way it is. This healthy eating plan of yours is impossible for a regular person with kids, a job and a husband to do."

Well that really lays it on the line, doesn't it? That last paragraph puts it all out there and is the very reason that it is most important that you understand WHY you are doing this. You cannot simply force yourself to do things differently. You really have to know why you are doing it. Something deep inside of you must change in order for you to successfully carry out this plan. You have to adjust your attitude. Again, you will have to change your mind about what is and isn't food. This can only happen when you are really, really sick of being fat, sick and having no energy.

This can only happen when you are really, really tired of popping pills and drinking coffee or Red Bull all day every day to keep your eyes open at work. This can only happen when you are really, really sick of your heart racing and your joints aching, of headaches, yeast infections, lumpy breasts, menopausal night sweats, mood swings, etc.

When you are really, really sick of being really, really sick and tired, then you may be ready to change your mind about what is and is not food. Every day, three to five times a day, we all make a decision to either eat well, feeding our bodies correctly, or to eat junk, causing premature sickness and disease. When you really change your mind about what is and isn't food, there is no way that you will look back.

It will not matter that your spouse doesn't like it. It will not matter if your friends are angry. It will not matter if your children are irritated that they cannot eat junk all day like all of their friends are doing. You will absolutely know that what you are doing is the right thing to do because you will be skinny and fit and you will feel amazing. In six weeks you will have lost several pounds and your brain fog will have cleared. You will no longer be addicted to junk food. You will be energized and you will be sleeping well all night long. Your hearing, taste and smell will all markedly improve due to improved blood flow through your veins and arteries. You will feel more alive than you have since you were a child. Your joints will not ache, your health problems will be starting to clear up and you will have an incredible amount of energy and you will feel amazing. Never underestimate the power of good nutrition.

My response to the above argument is that taste is not completely biological, it is a learned behavior. Children the world over eat the diet that their parent's provide them with. Research done by parenting experts has recently discovered that in order for a child to be comfortable with a new food item, they may need that food item served to them up to seventeen times before they will willingly eat it. Parents today get so discouraged if the food isn't eaten the first or second time that it is served that they just give up. This ends with all of their children eating what is commonly referred to as the "white" diet of pizza, crackers, candy, bread, and juice with chocolate milk to drink, etc. When you come to think of it, isn't this the diet that all American's eat now? Isn't the standard American diet just a whole lot of white, refined, "candy carbohydrates", meat, cheese, yogurt and sweetened beverages that contain almost no real nutrition at all? Most people eat a diet of meat, eggs, cheese, candy, cookies, crackers, cakes and chips washed down with soda. That's it. That is what they eat. All day, every day.

As a country we allow all of the children to eat this way despite the fact that it is especially important to feed children properly as when you feed them you are building the foundation of a proper diet. Hopefully these children will consume this proper diet for the rest of their lives.

Children will crave comforting foods that they associate with being cared for by their parents for their entire lives. It is so important to feed them properly from the beginning so that they grow up used to eating healthful foods. Children eat what their parent's eat. American's tend to want to eat white potato products covered in sour cream and milk, ice cream, macaroni and cheese, fried chicken, white bread spread with butter, cartons of yogurt, chips, crackers and canned vegetables because that is how they were raised. American's crave these foods because those are the foods they enjoyed as children. These are the foods that they associate with comfort and familiarity.

When you first begin to eat healthfully, you should do your best to make healthier versions of the foods that you enjoyed previously and change them over either gradually or all at once. To make these typical meals into healthier versions, a family might change from white rice to brown rice or blended multigrain rice and add more vegetables to stir fry dishes. Other easy fixes are to stop cooking with oil and stop adding excessive salt. It is quite possible to make and enjoy mashed potatoes made with vegetable broth and nutritional yeast with mushroom gravy and some type of meat analog product while the family gets used to eating a better diet. White bread and butter can be changed into wheat bread and low sugar strawberry jam. Macaroni and cheese can be replaced with whole grain macaroni and NOT cheese (see recipe section), plenty of steamed greens prepared healthfully and vegetarian riblets and vegan "chicken" patties can replace the previous favorites. The meat analog products are not as healthy as eating whole grains and vegetables but do help people accept the changes to their diet in a slow and steady way.

Changing the diet of your family and yourself will not be easy because it will be change but the results of improved health and a slimmer waistline will make it all completely worth it. This does not mean you cannot ever enjoy eating your previous favorite foods again. It is possible to enjoy "festival" days, perhaps five to ten important holidays a year, in which you can indulge in your usual favorites without worrying. But if it is not your birthday, and it is not the fourth of July, Christmas, or any other important holiday, stop eating like it is. With that being said, I have found that trying to eat those foods after eating very healthfully for long periods of time, just causes me to feel ill. This feeling is familiar, as I used to feel that way all of the time and I find that it is simply not worth it. I like to be healthy and feel good all of the time.

I like to compare eating healthfully to moving to a new country. At first everything is strange and different and it can be difficult to find anything to eat that you enjoy. But after you have been in the country for a while, you began to have your new favorite foods. After a while you begin to look forward to your new favorites. Most households eat the same seven to nine suppers and just rotate them regularly. If you come up with several recipes that you enjoy that are made out of very nutritious foods, then the change will not be as difficult and you and your children and spouse will look forward to eating delicious and nutritious meals. And the best part of all of this is that you will be much healthier and as a result of your new found health you will be much happier.

I believe that change is possible; it is difficult because it is change but with the right mental state and proper preparation, it is possible. When you change the way that you eat, at first everything will taste funny and be different. There are ways to make change easier. You have to decide if you are the kind of person who jumps into the pool or if you are the kind of person who gently wades in over twenty minutes or so. The person who jumps in will have the fastest results and will begin to feel better, faster, skinnier and healthier almost immediately (One to two weeks). The person who wades in slowly will continue changing one thing at a time, following the steps slowly and carefully, and will begin to feel better in one to two months and look a lot better and have more energy after about six months. It is up to you to decide which plan you would like to implement. I am usually a wade into the pool kind of person myself but after suffering from body aches and eczema for so long I will admit that I jumped into healthful eating with both feet and haven't looked back at all. The results of my diet change were nearly immediate and stunning and very fast as were my husband's.

Either of these methods will eventually bring you to the goal of excellent health through good nutrition and exercise. Remember that this is not a diet, it is a live it. This is the way you will live for the rest of your life. These changes are permanent changes to your lifestyle.

I believe that you can change the way that you eat and that your taste buds will change with you. Please understand that this change requires that you have the right attitude. The body does have to be re-set. It is worth it to note that the craving for fatty foods usually lasts about eight to ten weeks. At first you may feel that something is "missing" from all of your food, and it is…the fat will be missing. When the fat is eaten, it triggers the dopamine receptors in the brains reward center, causing a chemical reaction that rewards you for eating fat. When I cook pancakes or muffins for people who are not used to eating healthfully, they always say that the pancakes or waffles taste good but would taste even better with a pat of butter or cream cheese on them. Eating without added fat can take some getting used to. This craving for fat is tied to our evolutionary history and this craving protected us from starvation when times were lean. Those who had eaten the most fat were better able to make it through lean times. Because eating fat causes more dopamine to be released into the brain it can cause us to get a "bump" of good feeling every time it is consumed. That is why ice cream can be such a comfort food. It has both sugar and fat. When you stop eating fat on everything, you will miss it at first. Your brain will be asking for its reward when these foods are eaten. The real reward will be when you look in the mirror. You may not even know that the fat and or excessive sugar is missing from your food but your body will. The craving for junk will be there. Just like a junkie looking for the next "high" your brain has been conditioned to expect its dopamine "hit" when you eat junk. Like I said, this craving may last eight to ten weeks and then it will diminish. Be understanding and patient with yourself as you go through this change. It is a good thing. This is a process but it is well worth the effort. You are worth it and the way that you feel when you eat well and exercise, there is simply no replacement for that.

As long as your pantry is well stocked with healthful ingredients, you do not have to plan your menu out in advance. If you like to plan this out and do that sort of thing, it will be easy to do, but if, like me, you like to just fix what is easy to do and tastes good and that you are in the mood for, as long as the staples are on hand you should be able to fix healthy, easy and nutritious meals without any difficulty.

Keep in mind that for the first three to four days that you are eating healthfully, you may feel a little ill as your body goes through a normal detoxification process. Be patient with yourself as you are detoxing from junk food. It should not last longer than that and then you will feel much better. In fact, you will start to feel REALLY GOOD! If you continue to feel ill past the first three to four days, make sure that you are eating enough calories. Often a person eating junk does not realize that they have been taking in an enormous amount of junk food calories. Many people eat copious amount of refined oil products all day long and don't realize that these oils, that they cannot even see, add four to seven hundred calories a day easily to the average person's menu. Real food contains a lot of very filling fiber. Many people who have tried to eat this way say that they feel weak. They simply need to eat MORE. They are not used to having to eat so much. If you notice that you feel weak, add more food to your diet.

Eating real food requires that you spend a lot of time chewing. This can be a strange sensation at first as most manufactured food items are deliberately made to "melt away" in the mouth and be very easy to chew up and swallow so that even more of them can be consumed in a shorter period of time. Junk food is literally manufactured to remove the need to chew so that large quantities can be eaten quickly. The more junk food that you eat, the more money the junk food companies can make. This is just business. Real food requires a lot of chewing.

When my parents came to visit me and I made them a taco salad with lettuce, refried beans, tomatoes, green onions and salsa, it took them forever to eat it as they are not used to eating food that requires so much chewing. Your jaws can even ache a little from all of the chewing that is necessary.

When you start eating healthfully, make sure that you are eating enough food. If you continue to feel ill after the fourth day or if you are taking any prescription medications at all, consult your physician, making sure to mention that you are now eating very healthfully. The reason for this is that most prescription medications are being given for conditions that are caused by eating garbage all day every day. When a person stops eating garbage, the need for these medications quickly vanishes, and the medications themselves can make you very ill if they are no longer needed. Remember to work closely with your physician to adjust your medications while you convert to a healthful eating plan.

I will use blood pressure medication as an example. When you eat high fat, salty junk food, including caffeine, meat, eggs, dairy, added oils and processed foods, the blood vessels in your body constrict, or become smaller, because the insides of the vessels are filled with fat and the dehydration from all of the salt makes the blood vessels smaller on the inside. Think about going to visit a person who is a hoarder. All of the junk that is in their house makes it difficult to walk around inside. Everything is disorganized and there are piles of junk literally everywhere.

Think of yourself as the blood trying to flow through these clogged arteries. You have to squeeze through narrow places and navigate carefully through this mess. This will definitely slow your progress through the house and it will definitely cause you to neglect certain areas of the house as there is just too much junk contained in some areas for you to even visit. This is how it is inside of your arteries when you eat a terrible diet. The blood in your body has to pump through narrowed arteries that are lined with fat. The blood is also thickened due to chronic dehydration and excessive fat intake and does not flow as well. So not only is the blood vessel tight and narrow as it is clogged with fat, the blood is also thick, due to dehydration and fat. Is it any wonder that half of all men in their forties have difficulty with erectile dysfunction and those just a little older often need hearing aides? The arteries in the penis are very small and these arteries, along with the ones in the inner ear, are often affected by artery disease long before the rest of their bodies are. Getting older doesn't inevitably include becoming hard of hearing and having erectile dysfunction. These two diseases are related to artery disease and just show up sooner because of how small the blood vessels are that lead to them.

When a person is given blood pressure medicine, often the medicine acts on the walls of the blood vessels, relaxing them open so that the thickened blood can flow through the narrowed arteries better, thus reducing the pressure inside of the blood vessels. The medication doesn't really fix the reason why the blood pressure was so high in the first place; it simply forces the blood vessels to be relaxed open and wider, allowing the thickened blood to more easily flow through the now widened vessels.

When a person eats a healthy diet, within just a few days, the dehydration is resolved with the intake of plenty of water from both the water that is now being consumed by the glassful as well as the water in the natural food items that are now being eaten, and the excess salt and fat is no longer present as manufactured junk food is no longer being eaten. This causes the blood to thin out and then the artery walls start to clear the excessive fat and this causes the blood to pump through the now cleaner arteries much more efficiently. It is like a huge dumpster just pulled up to the hoarder's house and all of the junk that was inside is coming out. As a result of this, the blood may "pool" momentarily in the now wide open blood vessels and as a result of this happening a person taking blood pressure medication will begin to feel ill and dizzy. Their medication will still be causing the blood vessel walls to relax, which is no longer necessary, and the medication will have to be adjusted as soon as possible so the person doesn't feel ill or faint. The problem the medication was meant to resolve will have been fixed by eating a proper diet.

I have also spoken to several people who say that they tried to eat like this on a previous occasion but had to stop as they were feeling ill. Again, my first question would be, did they eat enough? It can take a lot of real food with very large portions to properly fuel the human body, especially one that is working hard to repair the damage caused by years of abuse and eating all of the wrong things. It is very important to listen to your body and eat enough calories. Remember that when you start eating correctly, everything else in your body will start to improve. You will definitely notice changes in your skin, hair and nails. There will be hormonal affects and changes.

Please do not be afraid to contact your physician with any and all concerns that you have about eating healthfully, especially if you are being treated for some kind of chronic condition. Making sure that you eat enough food is very important. Again, just to re-emphasize this point, there is not a single nutrient in meat, dairy and eggs that cannot better be supplied to the body in vegetables, whole grains, fruit, beans and nuts /seeds. The only supplement that you need to take is Vitamin B12 and possibly Vitamin D if you never go outside or live in a cold climate. That is it. The reason that you will need to take Vitamin B12 is because it is the only nutrient that is not found in today's vegetables. Vitamin B12 is produced by bacteria. Meat is covered in bacteria so the vitamin B12 is present in animal products. When we consume animals or animal products, we obtain the Vitamin B12 that we need by eating the animal flesh. We also used to obtain vitamin B12 by eating produce that had been grown in dirt and then not been washed and by drinking bacteria laden ground or well water. Now we have clear, running water and we always wash our vegetables and fruits, thus washing off any bacteria that might be producing Vitamin B 12 for us before we eat it. I personally would like to continue washing my vegetables and drinking clean water so I will just take Vitamin B12 supplements a couple of days a week and have no worries about it. A six month supply is really inexpensive. Supposedly, you have enough vitamin B12 in your body already to last for several years and it is not possible for any vitamin deficiency to show up in a short period of time, but I would rather ere on the side of caution and for that reason I will just take supplemental Vitamin B12 and again, not worry about it.

Other diet plans seem at first to be similar to my plan in that they claim to be very healthy and natural. The difference is that this plan is healthy, natural and EASY. The emphasis on easy is necessary because the list of ingredients and the complicated recipes of many of the diet plans that are similar just make them impossible for someone like me, and possibly you, to do. Not only that, they tend to contain large amounts of animal protein and added fat. The idea behind the Skinny and Fit but Never Hungry a Bit plan is to limit animal foods such as meat, dairy and eggs, if eaten at all, to just one to two servings per month, while increasing a person's intake of foods that are known to be much healthier including vegetables, fruits, whole grains, beans, nuts and seeds considerably. Added fat of any kind has been shown to be detrimental to heart health. The best kind of fat is the kind that doesn't get eaten! Like Dr. John McDougall says, "The fat you eat IS the fat you wear", either in your arteries or on your waistline. Yes, I am aware that fat is necessary for the functioning of many organs and tissues but are you aware that all plant foods contain some fat? Even spinach has 0.1 grams of fat per 1 cup. Many fruits also contain small amounts of fat. Every plant there is has some small amount of fat, placed in the plant in the perfect ratio and in the perfect package that our bodies readily and easily know what to do with it.

Is This Healthy? Won't I get sick if I eat this way?

NO! You will be healthier than everyone else!

The amounts of fat in this plan are adequate for normal human growth, development and maintenance and are optimal for human health. For most individuals, this diet is much healthier than what they usually eat and will prevent and reverse many disease processes. This plan has enough nutrients to properly fuel a growing baby or child over the age of two. Of course breast milk is the best food for infants and toddlers. Please consult your pediatrician or read the book, "Disease Proof Your Child" by Dr. Joel Fuhrman for excellent advice on feeding infants, toddlers and children.

Skinny & Fit but Never Hungry a Bit

This book has been an attempt to take a very serious topic of obesity with its natural consequences, heart disease, Type II diabetes, hypertension, many forms of cancer and high cholesterol, and make it easier to understand the causes and the cures. In the end, the only thing that really matters is your health. If you have your health you can do anything. Heart disease, diabetes and many types of cancer and autoimmune disorders are all diseases related to lifestyle choices and it is not your fate to die prematurely from any of them no matter what your genes are. Following the advice in this book will lead you to permanent weight loss, improved health and very likely will add years to your lifespan.

It is my sincere hope that you will take this effort seriously. Some people will inevitably say that they would rather die earlier than eat healthfully most of the time and they cannot stand to eat fruit and vegetables. This plan is not about living forever as we all must die one day. It is about adding health and vitality to the years that we do live. Being overweight and sick with diseases and pathological states is not a very nice way to spend years and years of your life. In countries where people do not eat junk all day, people are usually well and healthy long into their eighties. They don't require diapers, walkers, and boatloads of pills to combat years and years of poor nutrition and health neglect. They don't spend their last years completely disabled and

242

uncomfortable. They are able to stay active and involved in their families and communities.

In our country we merely warehouse our older citizens until they succumb to their disease states that have been brought about by years of poor nutritional choices. A common cause of death in other countries where junk is not eaten all day every day is simply to fall asleep and not wake up, having gone to bed after having a normal day the day before. And by a normal day I mean, walking their grandchildren home from school, preparing meals, gardening, etc. Jack LaLanne, who was considered to be the first fitness superhero, represents an American who ate properly and exercised regularly, more regularly than this book or plan requires. He did his entire workout the day before he passed away at age ninety three. His life and death are a great example to all of us of what eating well and exercise can do.

If you follow this plan with great success and this book has helped you , please contact me and let me know of your success. I sincerely wish you all of the best.

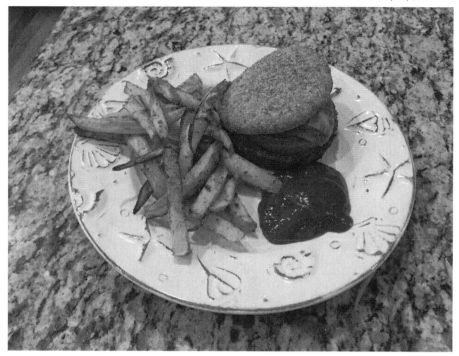

Chapter 7: Recipes

Meals and Snacks that Are Easy to Make and Easy to Live With

Ok. I will admit right here that I am no gourmet cook. The food ideas and recipes contained in this book represent tasty survival foods that can be put together quickly and appeal to most palates. There are many, many very good sources of vegan, whole food, plant based recipes with blogs and vlogs, websites and other books. These are simply fast ideas that work well for us working folks who do not have all day and night to spend in the kitchen cooking and then cleaning up a huge mess. These food ideas should get you through the week. Please feel free to alter them and come up with ways to make them your own. Most of these recipes are modified from unhealthy foods that I used to eat quite a lot of. They are my healthier versions. I know that in many cases there are even healthier options available but I am trying to appeal to the "real" people and not to the saints among us. I need food that I can actually eat and enjoy while I eat it. Maybe someday my tastes and my palate will become more sophisticated, but for now, these recipes represent what is fast and easy and tasty for me, and of course, most importantly, is healthy as well.

Keep it simple. Stick to the plan. Follow the rules. Remember on this plan there is no calorie counting, no limitations on healthy foods and no portion control. The only thing is that everything you eat must be the healthiest option that you can find at the time. With everything that you put in your mouth, think, "Is this healthy? Is this the best option I could eat right now?"

If the answer is no then don't eat it! Do not worry about "carbs" or carb counting or eating too many carbohydrates. The skinniest people in the world lived in Asia and Africa and all they ate were carbs. The difference was that they didn't eat a lot of meat, they ate almost no dairy products and they had minimal added oil and fat in their food. That is why they were so skinny! Times are changing as they adopt our western diet and they, too, are now getting sick and fat. You should stick to "good" carbs, like whole grains, beans and fruit and not bad ones like white bread, white sugar and most processed foods. Avoid excess sugar, salt and especially fat. Food manufacturers use cheap ingredients, add sugar, salt and / or fat in a high enough quantity and sell it as food for a profit. This is not food. This is garbage. Don't eat it! Do not ever go hungry. Have another piece of fruit, carrot sticks with hummus, pumpkin seeds, grapes, etc. Don't ever go hungry or you will be vulnerable to over eating bad food. Don't let this happen. Stay full of healthy food and you will find this to be easy.

Vegetable dishes can sometimes be bland especially if you are used to eating the "carnival" type food that most American's eat on a daily basis. Most dishes can be markedly improved by adding a little bit of salt and / or pepper after the cooking process, and I do mean a very little bit, just a sprinkle or two. Also a little bit of lemon juice, wine, beer, vinegar or vegetable broth can really help to improve the flavor of a dish. If you are making a dish that is based on one that used to contain cheese or dairy, topping it with a little "no cheesy sprinkle" can help a lot. Make sure you use the spices in your kitchen cupboard to dress your meals up and make them move flavorful. Don't be afraid to experiment. If you are not sure how something will taste, take a small amount of the food that you are preparing, set it aside and add a minuscule amount of spice and mix them together so that you can taste test it before adding the spice to your whole dish and possibly ruining the dish. Always remember to add a tiny bit at first. You can always add more but once put it in, you cannot get it back out again.

There is a flavor called "Umami" flavor that meat, dairy, eggs and milk impart into food that you may be very used to if you had previously been eating a meat heavy or meat centric diet. You can accomplish an Umami flavor in your vegetable and grain dishes by adding some glutamate to your dish. This can be accomplished by adding a few sprinkles of low sodium tamari or soy sauce. Don't add enough so that you can taste the tamari or soy or to flavor the dish, just adding a little bit will impart "Umami" flavor without adding enough to actually taste.

Toppings and Condiments that Are Nice to Have on Hand

In addition to the usual ketchup, barbecue sauce, etc. Here are a few special flavoring agents to keep in the refrigerator to help make your meals taste delicious.

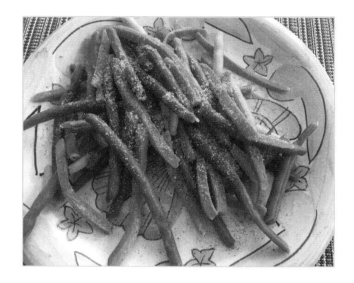

No Cheesy Sprinkle

Ingredients:

½ cup of unsalted raw cashews or almonds

½ cup of Nutritional Yeast

1 teaspoon of Mrs. Dash (optional)

1 teaspoon onion powder

Method:

Place all ingredients into a food processor. Process until it resembles Parmesan Cheese. Store it in a tightly closed container in the refrigerator. Use it on everything that needs "a little something", such as steamed vegetables, salads, pasta dishes, etc.

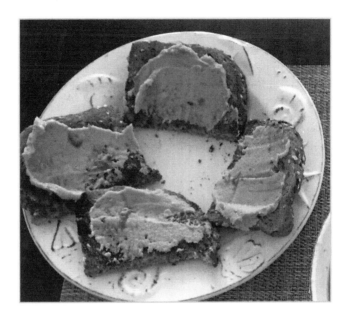

Red Pepper Lower Fat Hummus

Most of the hummus that you buy in the store is loaded with fat and is just about as bad for you as butter or margarine. You have to make your own in order to make sure it is truly healthy. If you decide to buy it, check the label to see how much fat is in the hummus. You can leave the red peppers out of this and change the spices around to suit your own taste but this particular one has a bit of a zing that I like.

15.5 ounce can of Garbanzo or any other kind of beans that you like

½ of a 4 ounce jar of roasted red peppers

1 / 8 cup of lemon juice or the juice from 1/2 lemon

1 clove of minced garlic or 1 tsp of bottled garlic

1 tsp. chipotle chili powder

½ tsp curry powder or turmeric

1 – 2 tsp sweetener such as brown sugar, agave, etc. (optional)

½ tsp. salt (optional)

Combine all ingredients in a food processor and process for 1 minute. Scrape the bowl and process again until smooth, another 1 -2 minutes.

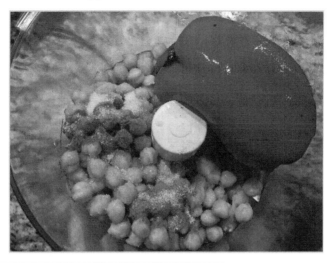

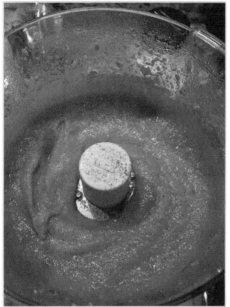

Sweet and Spicy Sriracha Hummus

Ingredients:

1 can of chickpeas, drained and rinsed well

1 bottled red roasted pepper, drained

Juice from 1/2 lemon

1 teaspoon bottled roasted garlic (or 1 garlic clove)

1 teaspoon chipotle chili powder

1 teaspoon Sriracha Sauce

1 teaspoon curry powder

1-2 teaspoons any kind of sweetener (sugar, brown sugar, maple syrup, agave nectar, etc)

1/2 teaspoon salt (optional)

Method:

Place all ingredients into a food processor, process thoroughly for 1 minute, scrape the sides of the bowl and process again for 1 - 2 minutes. Adjust seasonings as needed.

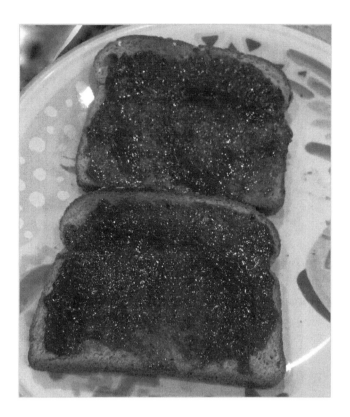

Low Sugar Strawberry Freezer Jam

This is absolutely delicious. You will never eat store bought jam again after tasting this.

Ingredients:

4 cups of crushed strawberries or other fruit, frozen or fresh to equal 4 cups exactly

3 cups of sugar

1 box of low sugar Sure-Jell or Certo fruit pectin

Method:

You will need to have 5 - 6 small (1 cup) freezer containers with lids. Make sure they are clean by washing them in hot soapy water and rinsing them. Crush the fruit and make sure you have exactly 4 cups of it, placing the measured fruit into a large, heat proof bowl. The directions on the Sure Jell box say to leave little pieces of fruit present to make jam but I am so lazy that I just take the frozen fruit out of the freezer, open the bag, pour it in a large heat proof bowl and let it defrost for several hours on the counter. I then puree the fruit in a food processor, measuring it out until I have exactly 4 cups, again, placed in the heat proof bowl. Then you place the 3 cups of sugar in a large saucepan and add the envelope of fruit pectin and 1 cup of water. Heat this up, stirring constantly, until it is boiling. Boil for one minute and then immediately pour this into the prepared fruit. Stir this for a few minutes and then pour it into the already prepared containers. Cover the containers and allow them to sit on the kitchen counter for 24 hours. Then put one container in the refrigerator and the rest in the freezer and enjoy.

Breakfast Ideas:

I try to keep this pretty simple. I am just not that creative with this stuff. I like to eat hot cereal, cold cereal, toast and / or fruit or smoothies on weekday mornings. On weekends, when you have a bit more time, you can get creative but the most important thing is to remember to just eat breakfast.

<u>Hot Cereal</u>

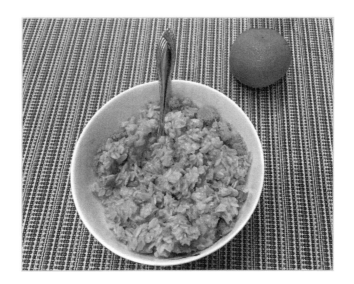

Oatmeal

Serves 1

Ingredients:

1 cup of old fashioned rolled oats

1 ½ cups of water

Pinch of salt

Pinch of cinnamon (optional)

1 – 2 teaspoons of sugar or other sweetener (optional)

1 Tablespoon of chopped nuts, or dates (optional)

¼ cup of fresh fruit (optional)

Method:

Place the water in a small saucepan, add a pinch of salt. Allow this to come to a full boil. Pour in the oatmeal, stirring constantly. Turn the heat to low and allow this to gently boil for 5 minutes. Add optional ingredients and serve with plant based milk.

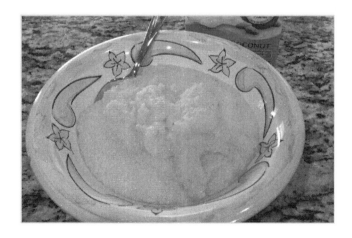

Corn Grits

Serves 1

Ingredients:

1/2 cup of yellow corn grits

1 ½ cups of water

Pinch of salt

1 – 2 teaspoons of sugar or other sweetener (optional)

Method:

Place the water in a small saucepan, add a pinch of salt. Allow this to come to a full boil. Pour in the corn grits, stirring constantly to avoid lumpy grits, a whisk works well. Turn the heat to low and allow this to gently boil, stirring intermittently for 5 - 8 minutes. Add optional ingredients and serve with plant based milk. You can also serve this with tofu scramble or a meat analog product, like a veggie sausage, without the added sweetener, for a savory breakfast.

Whole Grain Toast

1 – 2 pieces of whole grain bread

2 -3 Tablespoons of freshly ground peanut butter

2 – 3 Tablespoons of Low Sugar Freezer Jam

Toast the bread, spread with peanut butter or jam.

<u>Nature's Bakery Fig Bars</u>

These come in many flavors and appear to be one of the only healthier options available for eating on the run. Any brand will work but this one has whole grains and less than 20 percent of the calories coming from added fat. When selecting bars to eat on the go you should look for whole grains and no trans fats with oil accounting for less than twenty percent of the calories . Enjoy a package of these along with a couple of pieces of whole, fresh fruit for a fast, on the go type of breakfast.

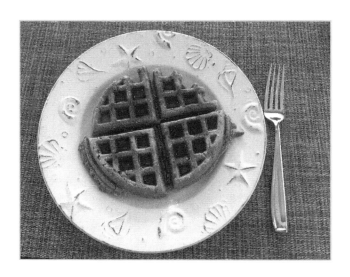

Waffles

Yield: About 8 waffles

Now this is something you can put together on a long, lazy weekend morning. If you make enough of them, you can refrigerator or freeze the leftovers so that you can enjoy them on work or school days as well. If you use a ceramic waffle maker you likely will not need to use non stick spray on the waffle iron but if you do not have a ceramic waffle iron you will probably not be able to keep these from sticking to the waffle iron without spraying it lightly with cooking oil spray. I do not use added fats or oils in cooking but to make waffles, I did use the nonstick spray until I bought a ceramic waffle iron. If you have heart disease, skip this recipe and stick to those that do not use nuts or nonstick spray.

Ingredients:

1/4 to 1/2 cup walnuts or pecans

1 Tablespoon of ground flax seed meal or chia seeds

3 Tablespoons of water

1 teaspoon of vinegar

½ cup of unsweetened apple sauce

1 1/2 to 2 cups of almond milk, almond / coconut milk, soy milk or any other plant based milk

1 teaspoon of vanilla

1 – 2 ripe bananas or ½ cup of pumpkin (optional)

1 cup of old fashioned rolled oats (optional, if not using, increase the flour by ½ cup)

1 1/2 cup of white or regular whole wheat flour

1 - 2 Tablespoons of brown or regular sugar or other sweetener (optional)

1 teaspoon of baking soda

1 teaspoon of baking powder

½ teaspoon of salt

½ - 1 teaspoon of cinnamon

Method:

Place the applesauce, the flax seed meal or chia seeds, water and plant based milk in a small bowl. Mix to combine and set aside for at least 5 minutes to allow the flaxseed meal or chia seeds to "gel" with the liquids.

Place the nuts in a food processor or high speed blender and pulse until finely chopped but not crushed. Place the nuts into a large mixing bowl.

Then place the oatmeal in the food processor and process it until it is finely ground.

Then mix the rest of the dry ingredients, including the rolled oats, flour, sugar, baking soda, baking powder, salt and cinnamon together in the food processor or blender and then add this to the large bowl with the nuts.

Then, place all of the wet ingredients, including the chia seeds or flax seed meal, vinegar, applesauce, vanilla, plant based milk and bananas or pumpkin if used into the food processor or blender and combine thoroughly.

Then add the wet ingredients to the dry ingredients in the bowl. Stir gently to combine; adding more milk if needed to make it the right consistency for waffles. Avoid over mixing or you will toughen the batter.

Lightly spray a waffle iron with no stick spray, or use a non-stick or ceramic waffle maker and place ½ cup of waffle mix onto waffle iron and close the lid. Remove the waffle when the indicator light on the waffle iron turns on saying that the waffle is finished cooking and enjoy with fresh fruit, organic maple syrup or low sugar jam or peanut butter.

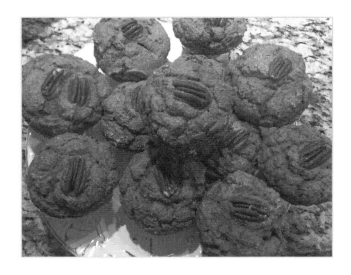

No Muffin Top Muffins

Yield: 12 Muffins

Again, this recipe is probably best utilized on the weekends or when you have extra time. I would like to say you can save some for breakfast throughout the week but they seldom last a day at my house.

Ingredients:

1 -2 Tablespoon of flax seed meal or chia seeds

3 Tablespoons of water

½ cup of unsweetened applesauce

2 cups of white or regular whole wheat flour, can be pastry flour

½ teaspoon salt

1 teaspoon baking soda,

½ teaspoon baking powder

2 Tablespoons to ¾ cup of sugar depending on how sweet you want them (optional), plus extra for dusting the tops prior to baking (optional)

1 Tablespoon of vinegar

1 cup of plant based milk

Any of the Optional Ingredients

Method:

Preheat the oven to 350 degrees.

Lightly spray a muffin pan with non – stick cooking spray, or use foil muffin tin liners. I have not had any luck using the silicone bakeware as it always makes the muffins have a plastic aftertaste and I end up throwing them all away. You can't use paper liners as these muffins have such a low amount of fat that they stick to the paper liners.

In a small mixing bowl, mix together the chia seeds or flax seed meal, 3 Tablespoons of water and the ½ cup unsweetened applesauce and set aside for at least 5 minutes to thicken.

In a large mixing bowl, place the whole wheat flour, salt, baking soda, baking powder, sugar, if added, and mix thoroughly to combine.

Add the vinegar to the plant based milk in the measuring cup and after mixing this, add it to the chia seeds or flax seed meal and apple sauce mixture in the small bowl. Combine all of the wet ingredients thoroughly.

Add the wet ingredients to the dry gently stirring as little as possible to avoid toughening the muffins.

Gently fold in any optional ingredients, if using.

Fill muffin cups 2 / 3 full and sprinkle muffin tops lightly with sugar or powdered sugar (optional). Top each muffin with a whole walnut or pecan (optional).

Bake the muffins for 18-22 minutes at 350 degrees until the muffin springs back lightly when pressed, or a table knife inserted into the center of a muffin comes out clean.

Optional Ingredients for different flavors:

For Apple Cinnamon Muffins, add 1 teaspoon of cinnamon to the dry ingredients and fold in 1 finely diced apple to the mixture just after combining wet and dry ingredients.

For Pumpkin Muffins: add 1 teaspoon of pumpkin pie spice to the dry ingredients and 3/4 cup of pureed canned or fresh cooked pumpkin to the wet ingredients.

For Banana Nut Muffins: add 1 teaspoon of cinnamon and ½ cup of chopped nuts to the dry ingredients and substitute a ripe banana for the applesauce

For Very Berry Muffins: Gently fold in ½ cup of chopped fresh or frozen berries to the muffin mix right after combining the wet and dry ingredients.

For double chocolate muffins, use ½ cup sugar and add 1/4 cup of cocoa powder to the dry ingredients and 1 teaspoon of vanilla to the wet ingredients. Gently fold in 1/3 cup of vegan chocolate chips, mini or regular size, to the batter after combining the wet and dry ingredients. Lightly dust the tops with powdered sugar after they finish baking.

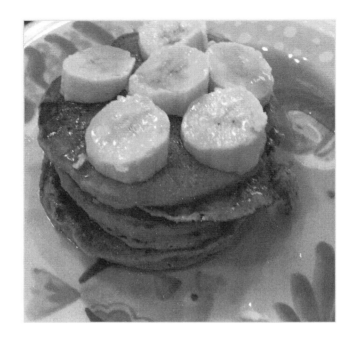

Healthy, No Egg, No Oil, No Dairy Pancakes

Yields: About 12 three to four inch pancakes

Ingredients:

1 -2 Tablespoons of flaxseed meal or chia seeds

3 Tablespoons of Water

½ cup of unsweetened applesauce

2 cups of white or regular whole wheat flour

½ teaspoon salt

1 teaspoon baking soda

1/2 teaspoon baking powder

1 Tablespoon sugar (optional)

1 ½ cups to 2 cups of plant based milk

1 Tablespoon of vinegar

Method:

In a small mixing bowl, mix together the chia or ground flax seeds, 3 Tablespoons of water and the ½ cup unsweetened applesauce and set aside for at least 5 minutes to thicken.

In a large mixing bowl, place the whole wheat flour, salt, baking soda, sugar, if using and mix the dry ingredients thoroughly to combine.

Add the vinegar to the plant based milk in the measuring cup and after mixing these two together, add this mixture to the chia or flaxseed meal and apple sauce mixture in the small bowl. Combine the wet ingredients thoroughly.

Add the wet ingredients to the dry ingredients, gently stirring as little as possible to avoid toughening the pancakes. Add extra plant based milk if necessary to get the right consistency for pancakes. The batter should be slightly lumpy but thin and easily pourable.

Ladle this out onto a hot non-stick griddle using a 1/3 cup measuring cup.

Be patient. When there are several bubbles on the pancake and the edges start to look a little dry, flip them over and cook the other side. Enjoy these pancakes with organic real maple syrup, homemade freezer jam, bananas, other fruit or peanut or other nut butters.

Optional Ingredients for different flavors:

Chocolate pancakes: Increase sugar to ½ cup and add 1/4 cup of cocoa powder to the dry ingredients and 1 teaspoon of vanilla to the wet ingredients. Gently fold in 1/3 cup of vegan chocolate chips, mini or regular size, to the batter after combining wet and dry ingredients. Lightly dust the tops with powdered sugar after they are finished cooking.

Apple cinnamon pancakes: Add 1 teaspoon of cinnamon to the dry ingredients. Fold in ½ cup of chopped apple to the pancake mix just before placing on the griddle.

Pumpkin pancakes: Use ½ cup of canned or pureed pumpkin instead of the applesauce in the wet ingredients and add 1 tsp of pumpkin pie spice to the dry ingredients.

Blueberry (or other fruit) pancakes: Fold in ½ cup of fruit to the pancake mix just before placing on the griddle.

Banana Nut pancakes: Substitute a ripe mashed banana for the applesauce. Fold in ¼ to ½ cup of chopped nuts just before placing on the griddle.

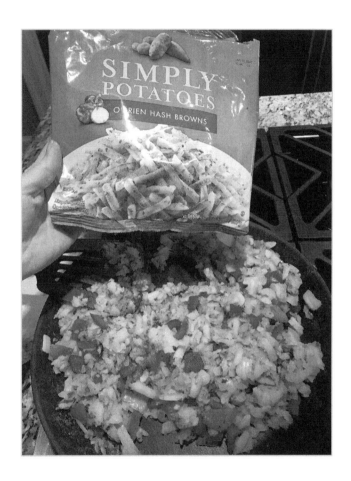

Hash Browned Potatoes

The easy way to do this is to go to the store and buy "Simply Potatoes" in the refrigerated case. I find these quite bland without the added oil so it is necessary to add about a half a chopped up onion and some bell peppers as well as some salt, pepper and / or Mrs. Dash, in any or all of her many varieties. You just cut open the bag of Simply Potatoes, place them in a non-stick skillet along with a chopped up onion and / or bell pepper and plenty of spices and keep cooking them while stirring intermittently for 12-15 minutes until you get some browning. Serve this with plenty of ketchup. You could also use a leftover baked potato and do the same thing. Or you could take a fresh potato, peel it and then grate it, cook it in the microwave for about 5 minutes and then place it in a non-stick skillet with the onion, bell pepper and spices.

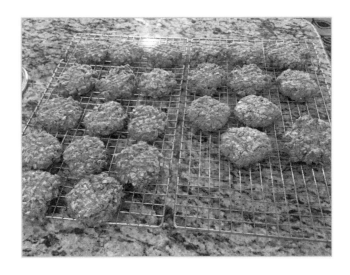

Suzanne's World Famous Breakfast Cookies

Yields: About 2 dozen cookies

Cookies for breakfast? Oh yes...I love cookies so much. When you are in a big hurry you can grab 1, 2, 3 or 4 of these for a great on the go breakfast. If your children play sports and you find yourself running all over the place with them, these are great for quick "pick me up" snacks. They are basically peanut butter, oatmeal, chocolate chip cookies. Instead of using butter, use nut butter. I cut the sugar down to a minimum that I could and still maintain a "cookie" like sweetness. Anyway, these are fantastic and you will love them.

Ingredients:

1 cup of natural, one ingredient peanut, almond or other nut butter

1 cup of brown sugar

1/2 cup unsweetened apple sauce, pumpkin or mashed banana

2 Tablespoons of Flaxseed meal

1/2 cup of plant based milk

2 teaspoons vanilla

2 cups rolled oats

1 1/2 cups of white or regular whole wheat flour

1 teaspoon baking powder

1/2 teaspoon baking soda

1/2 teaspoon salt

1/2 cup vegan mini chocolate chips or 1/2 cup chopped peanuts or other nuts (optional)

Method:

Preheat the oven to 350 degrees. Line 2 baking sheets with parchment paper.

Place the first 6 ingredients in a large mixing bowl and set aside to allow the flaxseed meal to "gel", about 5 minutes.

Place the rolled oats, flour, baking powder, baking soda and salt in a small mixing bowl and combine thoroughly.

Add the dry ingredients to the large bowl with the wet ingredients and combine thoroughly. Add in the mini chocolate chips, peanuts or other nuts if you like (optional).

Scoop out the dough onto the baking sheets 1 tablespoon at a time, form into a ball and flatten with a fork dipped in flour or sugar, like you would for peanut butter cookies. Bake for 12 - 14 minutes or until the edges start to lightly brown. Remove from the oven and allow to cool on the pan for 5 minutes before moving to a cooling rack. Makes about 2 dozen cookies.

<u>Lunch Ideas</u>

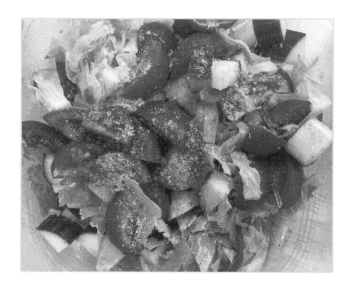

Garden Salad

Ingredients:

1 – 2 heads of romaine lettuce

8-12 cherry tomatoes or 1 large regular tomato

½ cucumber, peeled if desired and cut into slices or diced into cubes

½ cup matchstick sized or sliced carrots

1 cup or more of baby spinach leaves

½ bell pepper, any color, cut into strips and diced

2 Tablespoons or so of chopped red onion

Method:

Take the romaine lettuce and place it on the cutting board. Use a sharp knife to first remove the stem and then slice it like a loaf of bread and then slice it again from top to bottom so that you have nice bite sized pieces of lettuce. Place this lettuce and the baby spinach leaves into a salad spinner and wash the salad and spin it dry. Place the lettuce mix into large serving bowls and then add the rest of the ingredients on top of it. Sprinkle generously with "no cheesy" sprinkle or use balsamic vinegar or any other flavored vinegar that you like. If you must use salad dressing, try to choose fat free varieties and dip only the tines of the fork into the dressing to impart some flavor to the salad without a whole lot of added fat or chemical flavorings. You can also dress the salad with homemade low fat hummus, refried beans or regular beans.

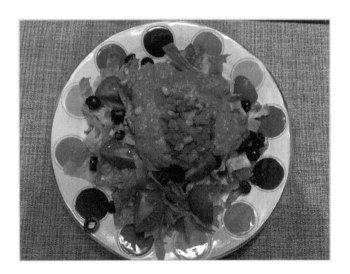

Suzanne's World Famous Taco Salad

Ingredients:

2 – 3 heads of Romaine Lettuce

1 can of vegetarian fat free refried beans

1 small can diced chilies

1 small can sliced black olives

6 – 8 cherry tomatoes

2- 3 green onions, sliced

Bottled or fresh salsa

Method:

Open the can of refried beans and the small can of chilies and place them both into a small saucepan. Combine them thoroughly and heat over low heat while you prepare the rest of the ingredients. Take the romaine lettuce and place it on the cutting board. Use a sharp knife to first remove the stem and then slice it like a loaf of bread and then slice it again from top to bottom so that you have nice bite sized pieces of lettuce. Place this lettuce into a salad spinner and wash the salad and spin it dry. Place the lettuce into large serving bowls and then top with the now heated refried beans / green chili combination. Then top with the rest of the ingredients. Add a few tablespoons of salsa and enjoy.

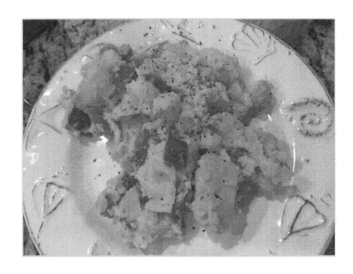

Potato Salad

Yields: 6 - 8 servings

Start with 6 – 8 large potatoes. Peel them, if desired, and then cut them into 1 inch cubes. Place them in a large saucepan, covering them with cold water. Bring them to a gentle boil over medium high heat. Allow to gently boil for 15 – 20 minutes or until fork tender but not mushy. Remove them from the heat, draining them into a large colander, rinse in cold water if desired or if you are in a hurry and then place them in a large bowl.

Also place into the bowl:

1 bell pepper, any color, sliced and diced

1 large cucumber, peeled, if desired, and diced

½ red onion, finely diced

4 – 6 green onions, finely sliced

2 – 4 stalks of celery, finely sliced and diced

Meanwhile, prepare the dressing for the potato salad:

1/2 cup water

1 cup of raw cashews

1/4 -1/2 cup raw cauliflower

Juice from 1 lemon

2-3 tablespoons yellow mustard

1 teaspoon sugar or other sweetener (agave nectar, maple syrup, etc) (optional)

1 tablespoon vinegar

1/2 to 1 teaspoon salt (optional)

Place all of these ingredients into a high speed blender. If you do not have a high speed blender, soak the cashews for 2 - 4 hours prior to making this recipe. Blend until smooth. Taste and adjust seasonings if necessary. Makes 1 1/3 cups of dressing.

Pour dressing over the rest of the potato salad ingredients in the large bowl, fold together gently to combine, adding salt and pepper as needed, refrigerate overnight or for several hours to allow the flavors to blend.

Cucumber Tomato Salad

Ingredients:

2 – 3 large tomatoes or 6 – 8 small tomatoes or 1 pint of cherry tomatoes cut into bite sized pieces

1 – 2 cucumbers, sliced thinly or thickly, as you desire

Place the tomatoes and cucumbers in a bowl and cover with

Cucumber Dill Salad Dressing:

2 tsp sugar or agave nectar

1/4 teaspoon salt

1/2 teaspoon dill

1/2 teaspoon parley

1/4 teaspoon pepper (white or black)

1 teaspoon mustard

Juice from 1/2 lemon

2-4 Tablespoons of Water

Method:

Combine thoroughly and pour over the tomato/ cucumber mixture. Refrigerate for a few hours to combine flavors

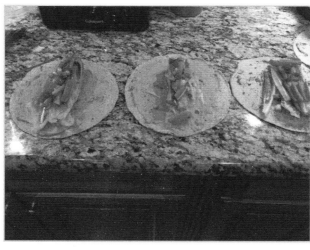

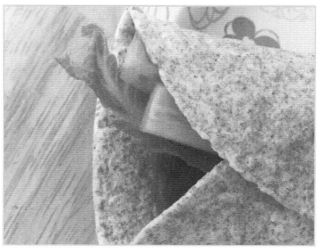

Vegetable Wrap

Ingredients:

Whole wheat tortilla

Romaine Lettuce

A few slices of red onion

Cucumber, skinned and cut into matchsticks

Bell Pepper, Sliced into thin strips

Prepared hummus

Method:

Take a whole wheat tortilla, spread with prepared low fat hummus.

Take a whole romaine lettuce leaf and place into the center of the wrap

Using the romaine lettuce as a base, add red onion, cucumber matchsticks and bell peppers.

Fold a small piece up from the bottom and then roll it tightly to make a sandwich wrap.

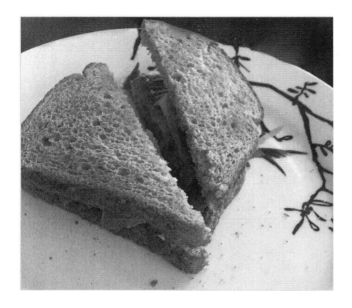

"Bacon" Lettuce and Tomato Sandwich

Ingredients:

2 slices of whole wheat bread, toasted

2 slices of some type of "veggie bacon", "cooked" in the microwave for 1 ½ minutes

Romaine lettuce leaf

2 – 3 slices of tomato

Method:

Place the romaine lettuce leaf on top of the toasted bread, top with veggie bacon and then the tomato slices and second slice of toasted bread. Cut in half and enjoy. If it seems too dry spread low fat hummus on the bread first.

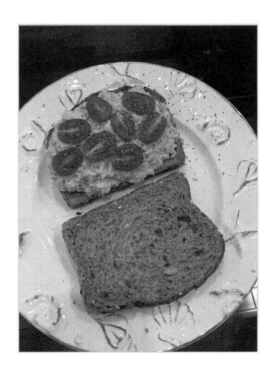

"Not Tuna" Salad

Sometimes you just want to eat a "tuna" sandwich. But of course fish is not a healthy option. This is a much healthier and, in my opinion, even tastier version.

Ingredients:

1 can of garbanzo beans, drained and rinsed

1/2 cup of raw, unsalted cashews

1/4 cup of water

2 teaspoon onion powder

1 tablespoon prepared mustard,

1/2 teaspoon salt

the juice from 1/2 lemon

1 Tablespoon of nutritional yeast

A few sweet pickles

If you do not have a Vitamix or high speed blender, soak the raw, unsalted cashews for 2 - 4 hours, then drain and proceed with the recipe. Place the beans in a medium sized bowl. Mash them with a fork or potato masher. Mix all of the rest of the ingredients together in a Vitamix or high speed blender for 1 minute. Then scrape down the sides and mix together again for 1 more minute. Pour over the mashed garbanzo beans and mix together until the mixture resembles tuna salad. Spread onto toasted whole grain bread and add some lettuce and / or slices of tomato and a pickle or two to complete the sandwich.

Soups

First I must say that making home made soup is so easy I cannot believe that we actually buy it in cans. Seriously. It is so easy. All you need to do is dice up a few vegetables, like celery and carrots and onions, let them brown a little in a big soup pot and then add all the rest of the ingredients and let it cook for a little while. Super easy. When I make soup, I really make soup. I enthusiastically cut up vegetables to the point where I need to use two large soup pots to contain all of the soup. When I am finished, I put some in the refrigerator to use during the next few days and I ladle the rest into freezer containers and place them in the freezer in single serving containers so I can quickly grab one on my way out the door in the morning for my lunch. Soup really comes down to the broth. You can make your own or you can buy broth. I buy low sodium vegetarian soup base that is concentrated. My preferred brand is "Better than Broth".

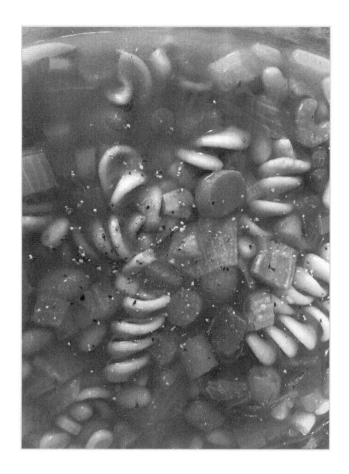

Minestrone Soup

My mom made this recipe for me. It is just delicious. I really cannot eat enough of it. Thank you Mom!!! When I make it I usually double or triple the ingredients so I will have plenty to freeze and save for later.

Ingredients:

1/2 cup navy beans, dried

in 1 cup of water

Bring this to a boil, then let sit for 1 hour.

After the hour, drain the beans and add:

6 cups of vegetable broth

2 cans of low sodium organic diced tomatoes

1 can of corn or 1/2 bag of frozen organic corn, drained and rinsed

4 sliced carrots

2 stalks of celery, sliced

1 diced onion

1 clove garlic

1 teaspoon basil

1/2 teaspoon salt

1/2 teaspoon pepper

Let this come to a boil and after 10 minutes or so add:

1/2 cup of whole grain pasta

Continue boiling for 10 - 15 minutes and its done!

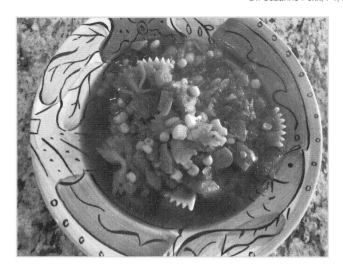

Vegetable Soup

Ingredients:

10 cups vegetable broth

1 large onion

3-4 carrots

3-4 stalks celery and leaves

2 cans diced low sodium tomatoes

1 cup or frozen organic corn

1/4 head of cabbage, sliced

1-2 cloves garlic

2 teaspoons basil

Pinch of sugar

1 1/2 cups whole wheat pasta, such as bowties

In a large soup pot dry sauté the diced onion until it is just starting to brown.

Add all the rest of the ingredients except the noodles. Bring to a simmer and let simmer for 20 minutes. Then add whole wheat pasta and let simmer for another 20 minutes. Enjoy.

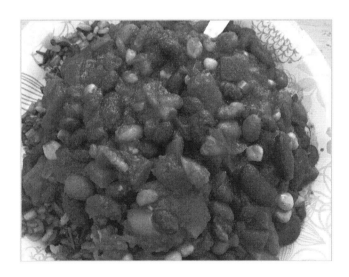

3 Bean Chili

Ingredients:

3 Bell peppers, any color, seeded and diced

1 large onion, diced

2 cloves of garlic or 2 tsp of bottled garlic

2 – 4 teaspoons chili powder

1 teaspoon cumin

¼ - ½ teaspoon ground black pepper

½ teaspoon smoked or regular paprika

¼ to ½ teaspoon cayenne pepper

2 14 oz cans low salt tomato sauce

2 14 oz cans low sodium diced tomatoes

1 can pinto beans

1 can kidney beans

1 can black beans

1 bag of frozen corn

1 Tablespoon brown sugar

Dash of cinnamon

Method:

Water sauté the peppers and onion in a large soup pot with 2 cloves of garlic until they are translucent.

Add 1 teaspoon cumin, 2 – 4 teaspoons of chili powder, ¼ - ½ teaspoon ground black pepper, ½ teaspoon of smoked paprika, ¼ to ½ teaspoon cayenne pepper. Stir to combine.

Then add 2 large cans of low salt tomato sauce, 2 cans of organic low sodium diced tomatoes.

Open the cans of beans and drain and rinse them into a strainer before adding them to the chili.

Place the corn into the strainer and rinse it under hot tap water to defrost it and then add this to the mixture.

Add 1 Tablespoon of brown sugar and a small sprinkle of cinnamon.

Let this all simmer for 30 minutes or so and serve over brown rice or with corn bread muffins.

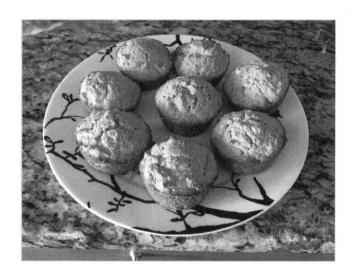

Corn Muffins

You can serve these corn muffins with the minestrone soup or the chili listed above. They are easy and delicious and most of all, will keep you skinny and fit!

Preheat the oven to 400 degrees. Prepare a muffin pan with foil baking cups.

Ingredients:

1 Tablespoon of Chia Seeds or 1 Tbsp of Ground Flaxseed Meal

3 Tablespoon of water

1/2 cup of unsweetened applesauce

1 cup of plant based milk

1 teaspoon vinegar

1/4 cup stone ground cornmeal

3/4 cup of regular or white whole wheat flour

1/4 to 1/2 cup of sugar

1 teaspoon baking powder

1 teaspoon corn starch (to soften the muffins, if you like them chewy, skip)

1/2 teaspoon baking soda

1/2 teaspoon salt

In a small mixing bowl combine the chia seeds or ground flaxseed meal, water, applesauce, plant based milk and vinegar. Set this aside to gel for at least 5 minutes. In a large mixing bowl, combine the cornmeal, flour, sugar, baking powder, corn starch, baking soda and salt. Make sure that the wet ingredients are mixed thoroughly and that the dry ingredients are also mixed thoroughly and then combine them together in the large bowl, mixing just until moistened. Do not over mix or the muffins will be tough. Spoon into prepared muffin cups and place in the oven for 18 - 20 minutes until a knife inserted into the center of a muffin comes out clean.

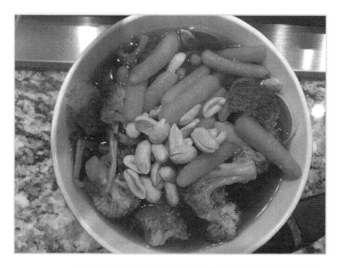

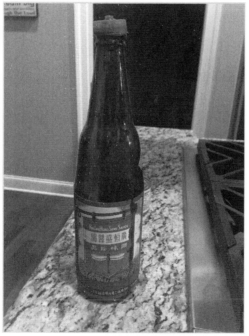

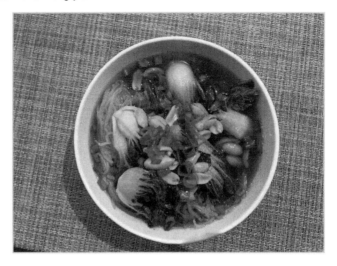

Thai Noodle Soup

My husband is from Thailand and when we were meat eaters this was a favorite soup of ours. It took a few tries for me to veganize it but I must say I like this version even better. The rice noodles are absolutely delicious. This is somewhat like Vietnamese "pho" type soups that are becoming widely available.

2 packages of rice noodles. Try to find the brown rice noodles but they are difficult to find. These rice noodles can be thin, thick, whatever you like. They are available at an asian grocery store.

The first step is to open the package of rice noodles and place the noodles into a large bowl and then cover them with water. Allow this to sit for 1 - 3 hours in water.

296

Then you make the Soup Base:

12 cups of vegetable broth

3 stalks of celery with leaves

1 onion, quartered

6 - 8 whole star anise

2 -3 cinnamon sticks

1/4 cup Kwong Hung Seng Sauce (also known as black soy sauce, should be thick like molasses. You can find this at an asian grocery store)

1 Tablespoon sugar

1 Tablespoon vinegar

Place all of the ingredients in a large pot and allow to gently simmer for 30 - 40 minutes, adjust seasonings to taste.

While this simmers, prepare the vegetables, any combination of 2 - 4 cups of broccoli, carrots, baby Bok Choy. Steam these in a pot separately for 10 - 15 minutes.

When the vegetables are done start another small pot of water boiling. When it is boiling, use a small hand held mesh strainer and place a handful of the softened noodles into the strainer basket. While holding on to the handle of the strainer, place the strainer basket into the boiling water using a chop stick to stir the noodles gently while they cook. The noodles will cook in 30 to 60 seconds. Pull them up out of the boiling water still in the strainer and let them drain for a few seconds and then place the cooked noodles into a large soup bowl. Add the steamed vegetables on top of the noodles. Then cover the noodles and the vegetables with the broth. Top the soup with fresh mint leaves, coriander leaves, Siracha sauce, vegetarian hoisin sauce, bean sprouts, chopped green onions and chopped peanuts. (All optional)

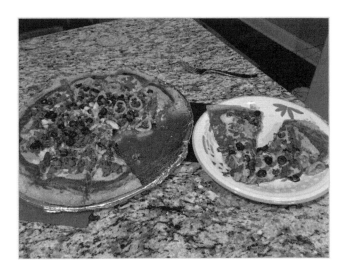

Pizza with homemade whole wheat no oil crust

Ingredients:

Pizza Crust:

1 pkg. quick acting yeast

2 – 3 cups of whole wheat or white whole wheat flour

½ to 1 teaspoon salt

1 / 2 cup of unsweetened applesauce

1 - 2 teaspoons onion powder

½ to 1 teaspoon of garlic powder

1 cup of warm water

Cornmeal to dust the pan with (optional)

Pizza Sauce:

1 14 oz can of no salt added tomato sauce

½ teaspoon pepper

1 – 2 teaspoon of garlic powder

½ - 1 teaspoons of sugar

2 teaspoons basil

2 teaspoons of Italian Seasoning

For the "Not Cheese" Sauce:

1 ½ cups cooked yellow corn grits

1 ½ cups of water

Dash of salt

1/3 to ½ cup of nutritional yeast

¼ cup raw unsalted cashews or canned cannellini beans

½ teaspoon salt

½ teaspoon pepper

1-2 teaspoons onion powder

1-2 teaspoons garlic powder

Pizza Toppings:

Sliced or Diced red onion

Sliced olives

Spinach, chopped

Sliced mushrooms

Sliced bell peppers

Anything else you like on pizza

Method:

Preheat the Oven to 400 degrees.

Prepare a pizza pan by spraying with no stick spray and then sprinkling with corn meal or use a pizza stone, silicone or parchment paper to avoid the non stick spray.

To prepare the pizza crust:

Combine the flour, the yeast and the salt, onion powder and garlic powder in a large bowl and mix thoroughly. Add the applesauce and warm water and mix until it like "dough". Knead it for a few minutes, adding extra flour as necessary until it forms a ball and then let it rest in the bowl covered with a moist paper towel for 10 minutes while you prepare the toppings.

After 10 minutes knead the dough again, using extra flour if necessary and let it rest again for 10 minutes, again covered with a moist paper towel.

After another ten minutes, roll the dough out with a rolling pin and shape the dough into a pizza crust and place it on a lightly sprayed pizza pan that has been lightly sprinkled with corn meal or on the parchment paper lined pan.

To Prepare the Pizza Sauce:

Place all of the ingredients for the sauce in a small saucepan and heat gently, stirring occasionally for 10 minutes or so.

To Prepare the "Not cheese" Sauce:

Cook the corn grits and then place all of the "cheese" ingredients into a high speed blender and blend for 2 minutes. It should look like cheese.

Top the crust with the "not cheese" sauce. Then spread the low fat pizza sauce on top and then add the toppings such as onions, spinach, mushrooms, olives, peppers, etc. Sprinkle with nutritional yeast and fresh or dried basil. You have to spread the "not cheese" sauce first as it has a thickened consistency and it is too difficult to spread on top of the tomato sauce.

Bake in a 400 degree oven for 18 – 20 minutes and enjoy!

Cook Out Ideas

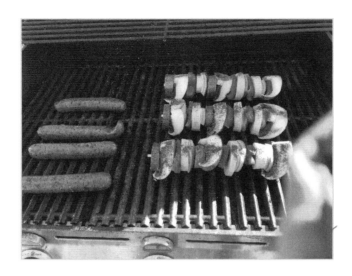

Buy vegan sausage, such as Tofurkey Italian Sausage and grill per the directions on a grill. Serve with whole wheat hot dog buns, sauerkraut, ketchup and mustard

Buy or make veggie burgers and serve with toasted whole wheat buns, "not cheese" sauce, pickles, sliced tomatoes, onions, ketchup and mustard

Veggie Kabobs

Slice onions, peppers, mushrooms and vegan sausages (optional) and thread onto kabob sticks, grill for 10 – 15 minutes turning halfway through. Serve with whole grain rice and beans for a hearty meal.

303

Corn on the cob

Wrap corn in foil and grill. There is no need to add oil or coat it with butter. Sprinkle with salt when it is finished.

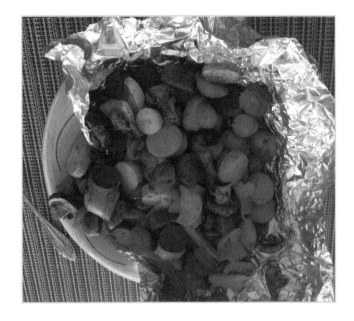

Grilled vegetables

Place cut up potatoes, onions, carrots and mushrooms and whatever kind of vegetables you like on a large piece of aluminum foil that has been lightly sprayed with no stick cooking spray. Sprinkle with Mrs. Dash, salt and pepper. You can also add a few slices of "Tofurkey" or other vegan sausage to this for extra flavor. Cover with additional aluminum foil to make a "package". Place on a grill and grill for about 1 hour. Serve with whole grain rice or mashed potatoes.

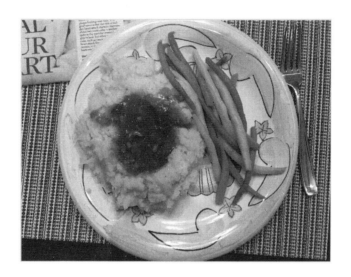

Mashed Potatoes

Ingredients:

8 – 9 Medium Sized potatoes

1 cup of vegetable broth made with potato water and low sodium vegetable soup base

2 Tablespoons of nutritional yeast

1 – 2 teaspoons of onion powder

½ to 1 teaspoons salt

¼ to ½ teaspoon pepper

Method:

Peel the potatoes (optional) and then dice them into cubes. Place in a saucepan and add water to cover them by ½ inch. Boil them for 20 minutes or until a fork pierces them easily.

Drain the potatoes in a strainer and then place into a large bowl.

Add the vegetable broth, nutritional yeast, onion powder, salt and pepper. Either use a hand mixer, stand mixer or a potato masher and mash them thoroughly. Adjust seasonings as needed.

Mushroom Gravy

Ingredients:

1 onion, finely chopped

½ pound of mushrooms, sliced

2 cups vegetable broth or leftover potato water

1 Tablespoon soy sauce or low sodium tamari sauce

2 Tablespoons of cornstarch

Method:

Water sauté the mushrooms and onion in a non stick skillet until the mushrooms are soft and the mushrooms release their liquids. Add 1 ½ cups of vegetable broth and soy sauce.

Add the 2 Tablespoons of corn starch to the last ½ cup of vegetable broth and mix this together thoroughly, with a fork or wire whisk.

Add this to the rest of the mixture, stirring constantly with a spatula. As it boils the gravy will thicken. It is finished when it has boiled for about 1 -2 minutes.

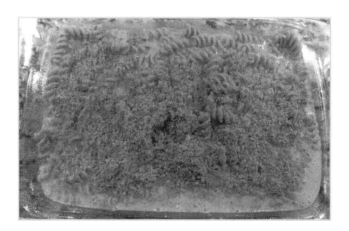

Macaroni and Not Cheese

Ingredients:

1 onion, diced

1/2 cup of raw unsalted cashews or canned white cannellini beans, rinsed and drained

1 1/2 cups of cooked yellow corn grits

Juice from 1 lemon or 1/3 cup lemon juice

2 cups water

1 tsp salt

2 - 3 roasted red peppers (optional)

1/2 cup nutritional yeast

1 tsp. garlic powder

2 tsp. onion powder

16 ounce box of whole grain elbow or rotini pasta

Method:

First, start a large pot of water boiling for the pasta, as this will take the longest.

Preheat the oven to 425 degrees

Line a large 9 x 13 baking dish with parchment paper.

Sauté the onion in a nonstick skillet until translucent, about 5 minutes

Place the cashews or cannellini beans, cooked onion, corn grits, lemon juice, water, and salt in a high speed blender or food processor for 1 minute or until well combined, then add the garlic powder, onion powder, nutritional yeast and roasted red peppers and blend thoroughly an additional 1 – 2 minutes.

Cook the pasta "al dente" and then drain it and place it back into the pot. Add the sauce from the high speed blender, stir to thoroughly combine and then place this into the prepared baking pan. Top with crushed croutons (croutons usually contain oil so leave these out if you are dealing with heart disease or have not reached your ideal weight yet) or whole wheat bread crumbs. Place in the oven and bake for 20 minutes until the top is lightly browned.

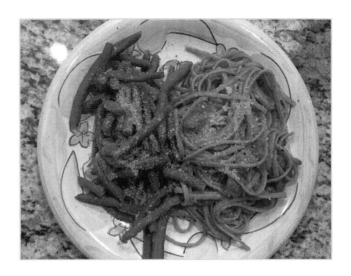

Spaghetti and Marinara Sauce

Look for low fat, low calorie marinara sauce (less than 25% of calories from fat) and serve over whole grain pasta. You can add sautéed mushrooms, onions, peppers and other vegetables to the marinara sauce to make it "chunky". You can add Tofurkey vegan sausage to this as well. Top with "no cheesy "sprinkle. Serve with steamed broccoli, peas or spinach. If you can't find a good marinara sauce you can make your own.

Ingredients:

1 Box of whole wheat pasta, spaghetti, thin or thick

1 diced onion (optional)

6 - 8 mushrooms, sliced (optional)

1 bell pepper, seeded and chopped (optional)

2 small zucchini, sliced(optional)

1 can low sodium organic tomato sauce

1/2 teaspoon oregano

1 teaspoon garlic powder

1 teaspoon onion powder

1 teaspoon basil

1 teaspoon Italian seasoning

1/2 teaspoons sugar or other sweetener (agave nectar, maple syrup)

Dash of cayenne pepper

Method:

Cook the whole wheat pasta according to package directions. Place the vegetables into a medium saucepan, if using. Dry sauté the vegetables for 5 minutes or so until the onion is translucent. Mix all of the other ingredients together and simmer for 5 - 10 minutes. Taste and adjust seasonings as needed. Enjoy!

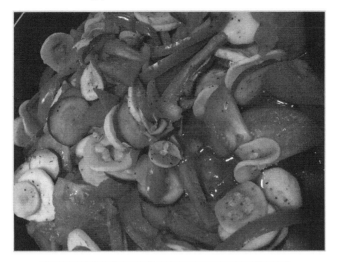

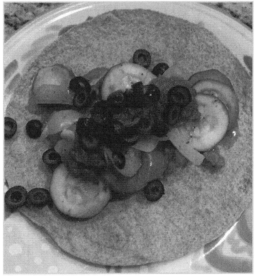

Fajitas

Ingredients:

2 - 3 sliced zucchini

2 -3 sliced yellow crook neck squash

1 to 1 1/2 cups sliced mushrooms

1 diced onion

1 - 2 sliced bell peppers, any color

1/2 - 1 cup fresh chopped tomatoes

In a large frying pain, dry sauté the onion until it begins to brown. Then add the rest of the vegetables and a small amount of water or low sodium vegetable broth or wine as necessary to keep the vegetables from sticking to the pan while they sauté. Usually the vegetables will release enough liquid that you can skip this step. Turn down the heat to medium low and cover the pan while you mix up the fajita sauce.

Fajita Sauce:

1 - 2 Tablespoons Corn Starch

2 teaspoons chili powder

1 teaspoon paprika

1 teaspoon sugar, or other sweetener such as agave nectar

2 teaspoons onion powder

1/2 teaspoon cayenne pepper

1/4 teaspoon black pepper

1 teaspoon ground cumin

Mix all of these in a small bowl and then, using a wire whisk or a fork, add 1 1/2 cups of low sodium vegetable broth to the spice mix. When it is mixed throughly, pour this over the top of the almost cooked vegetables and stir until the sauce boils and thickens. Cover while you heat up the refried beans and tortillas.

Serve by placing 1 tortilla on a plate after heating it in a large dry frying pan or in the microwave for 10 - 20 seconds, then add a line down the middle of fat free vegetarian refried beans, spoon on the fajita vegetables and sauce and then add some bottled or fresh salsa. Roll up the tortilla and enjoy.

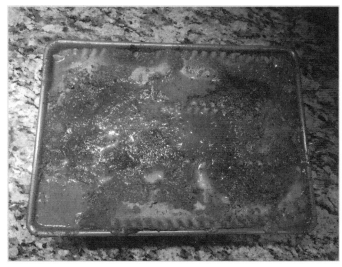

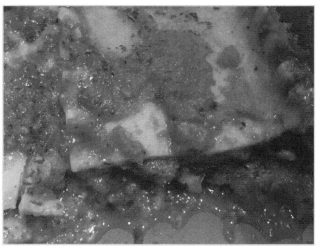

Vegetable Lasagna

Makes a 9 x 13 pan

Ingredients:

2 10-ounce packages frozen chopped spinach, OR 2 pounds fresh spinach, rinsed, chopped, and steamed

1 pound mushrooms, sliced (about 5 cups)

1 onion, finely diced

1 garlic cloves, thinly sliced

1 tablespoon soy sauce

2 tablespoons balsamic vinegar

3/4 teaspoon salt

1/4 teaspoon ground black pepper

1/4 teaspoon ground nutmeg

1 teaspoon garlic powder

1 teaspoon onion powder

1/4 cup raw unsalted cashews

1/2 cup corn grits

1/4 cup nutritional yeast

I roasted red pepper (optional)

25-ounce jar vegan marinara sauce or a prepared recipe of marinara sauce

10 - 12 dry (no boil) lasagna noodles (about 12 ounces)

Method:

If necessary, thaw the frozen spinach. If you do not have a high powered blender, such as a Vitamix, soak the cashews for 2 -4 hours before using then drain them and proceed with the recipe.

Preheat the oven to 350 degrees

Prepare a 9x13 pan by spraying with non stick spray or lining with parchment paper.

Prepare the corn grits in 1 1/2 cups of water according to package directions

Combine cooked corn grits with cashews, onion powder, garlic powder, nutmeg, nutritional yeast, roasted red pepper, black pepper, and salt in a high speed blender with 1 cup water.

Blend on high speed until completely smooth, about 2 minutes, stopping blender occasionally to scrape down sides with a rubber spatula. Set aside.

Heat vinegar, soy sauce in a large skillet. Add onion and garlic and cook 1 minute over medium-high heat, stirring constantly. Reduce heat to medium and add mushrooms. Cover and cook for about 5 minutes, stirring often, until browned.

Meanwhile, in a large pot, steam the minced fresh spinach for 5-8 minutes. Drain if necessary and Cook briefly over medium heat for 2 to 3 minutes, stirring often, to remove any excess moisture. Add the corn grits "no cheese" sauce mixture and cook for about 3 minutes, stirring frequently, until mixture thickens slightly. Remove from heat.

Spread 1 1/2 cups marinara in a 9"×13" baking dish. Top with a layer of noodles, slightly overlapping, and half of the mushrooms. Spread with half the spinach mixture and half the remaining marinara.

Repeat layers with remaining noodles, mushrooms, spinach, and marinara sauce. Cover with a sheet of baking parchment (this prevents contact between the tomato sauce and aluminum foil), then wrap tightly with aluminum foil.

Bake for about 1 hour, removing the foil after the first 30 minutes, until the noodles are tender (test by inserting a knife into the center of the lasagna). Allow the lasagna to stand uncovered for 15 minutes before serving.

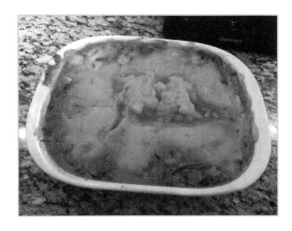

Shepherd's Pie

Makes a 9 by 13 inch baking dish.

Preheat the oven to 350 degrees. Prepare a 9 x 13 inch baking dish by spraying with no stick spray or lining with parchment paper.

Make mashed potatoes:

Peel 5-6 potatoes and then cut them into chunks. Place the potatoes into a large saucepan. Cover the potatoes with water. Boil 15-20 minutes until they are easily pierced with a fork. Drain, reserving 2 to 3 cups of the potato water. Mash the potatoes using the potato water, 1-2 teaspoons of onion powder, 1-2 teaspoons of salt and 1/2-1 teaspoon of white pepper. Add 1/4 - 1/2 cup of nutritional yeast to add richness. Mash them well. Add extra potato cooking water or seasonings as necessary until they are perfect.

Make vegetable mix:

Meanwhile, finely dice 1 or 2 onions, place in a large non stick frying pan that has been heated for a few minutes so that it is hot.   While the onions cook and lightly brown slice 4 stalks of celery and 4-6 large carrots.   Add to the onion and stir sauté, adding potato water as necessary to keep it from sticking.   Then add 3 cups of sliced green beans and 1 bag of frozen peas.   Allow this to heat thoroughly while you make the gravy.

Make gravy:

Place 4 cups of vegetable broth in a large saucepan.   Add 1-2 tsp of onion powder, 1-2 tsp of Herbs de Provence and 1-2 tsp of low sodium Lawrys seasoned salt.   Then place 4 - 6 tbsp of whole wheat flour into a liquid measuring cup.   Add cold water to cover and then whisk this to make it into a slurry.   Make sure that all of the flour is mixed in well.   Add this to the seasoned broth that is lightly boiling and continue stirring and bring to a boil once again to thicken the gravy.   Taste and adjust the seasonings if necessary.

Combine and bake:

When the gravy is perfect add the gravy on top of the vegetable mix, stir to combine and then pour into a 9 by 13 inch baking pan.   Cover the vegetables with the prepared mashed potatoes and place in a 350 degree oven for 45 minutes.

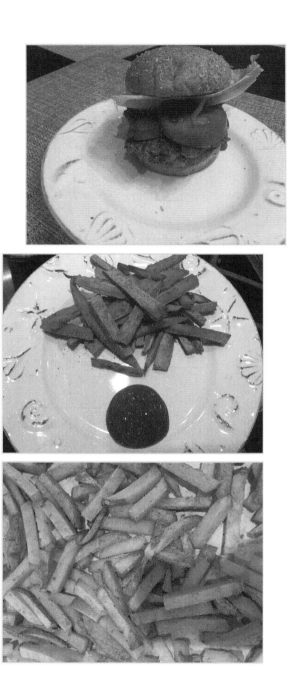

Burgers and Fries

Burgers with No Cow, No Oil and No Egg

The key to making a good veggie burger is ground flaxseed meal and enough moisture to make it all stick together while it cooks. You can use any combination of these type of ingredients that you like. Experiment and make this recipe your own.

Ingredients

1 can black beans, or any other kind

1 cup oatmeal (rolled, steel cut, doesn't matter)

2 tablespoons flax seed meal

2 teaspoon onion powder

1/2 to 1 teaspoon chipotle chili powder

1/2 teaspoon low sodium soy or Tamari sauce

1 bell pepper, seeded and chopped, any color

1 small onion, chopped

6 or so mushrooms

Method:

Drain the beans but don't rinse them. Mix all of these ingredients together in the food processor and set aside to "gel" while you prepare the vegetables.

Dice 1 bell pepper and a small onion, sauté in a dry pan until the onion softens and begins to turn light brown.

Add 6 or so finely chopped mushrooms. When this is cooked add this to the bean mixture and pulse several times in the food processor to mix thoroughly.

Scoop out 1/2 cup of mixture at a time and gently shape into a patty. Place in a nonstick pan to cook, after 3-5 minutes turn and lightly brown the second side.

Alternatively you can bake in the oven at 350 on parchment paper for 30 minutes and turn over after 15 minutes. Sooo good! You can try to grill these as well if you are feeling brave. Serve them on whole wheat buns with lettuce, tomato, ketchup, onions and whatever else you like.

Sweet Potato Fries

These are just delicious. I like to make them kind of spicy, but you can leave out the hot ingredients if you like. I have heard they will be even better if you cut up the fries and then soak them in water for at least one hour prior to making the fries. I never have had the time, but for you foodies, you might try it.

Preheat the oven to 425 degrees

Prepare 2 baking pans by lining with parchment paper

Ingredients:

3 sweet potatoes, peeled and chopped into "fry" shapes

1 tablespoon white whole wheat flour, 1 teaspoon of low sodium Lawry's seasoned salt

1 teaspoon chipotle chili powder

Dash of smoked or regular paprika

Dash of cayenne pepper

Method:

After you cut the sweet potatoes into fry shapes they will be slightly damp, place them in a large bowl. (If you have the time, soak them in water for at least 1 hour and then drain the water off. If you don't have the time, proceed, they just won't be as crispy).

In a smaller bowl, mix all of the spice ingredients together. Shake spice ingredients over the prepared potatoes and mix thoroughly. Spread evenly in a single layer on the baking pans and place in the oven. Bake at 425 for 30 minutes, or until they begin to brown. Halfway through the baking process, rotate the pans. After 30 minutes, turn off the oven and open the door a crack and let them sit in the oven for an additional 10 minutes. Serve with ketchup. Enjoy!

To make regular french fries you follow a similar recipe. I use either the recipe from "The Brand New Vegan" or from Will Kriski's website, "Potatostrong" and I highly recommend that you take a look at both of these websites for absolutely fantastic food ideas!

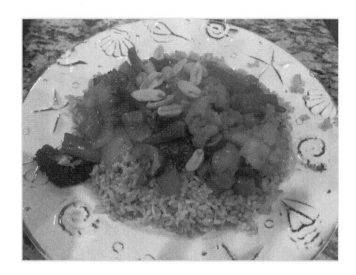

Vegetable Stir Fry with Peanuts

First, make whole grain rice.

The very best rice is brown jasmine rice. You can usually find this at an asian grocery store. You make the rice by rinsing 2 cups of rice and placing in a saucepan with a tight fitting lid or a rice cooker. Add 3 cups of water and a pinch of salt. Bring to a boil and then simmer for 45 minutes to 1 hour. Avoid opening the lid and don't stir this while it cooks or you will make it mushy. Just leave it alone and let it cook. If you use a rice cooker, place these ingredients in the rice cooker and push the button for brown rice. Another delicious rice is the rice blend, made of all different kinds of whole grain rice, red, brown, wild, etc. You make it the same way as the jasmine brown rice. You can also make regular brown rice using this same recipe and method. There is a quick cooking brown rice I found at Costco that cooks in the same time as white rice, 20 to 30 minutes. You cook it the same way as the above whole grain rice but it only takes 20 -30 minutes.

Ingredients:

1 onion, diced

1-2 teaspoon bottled garlic

4-6 cups of cut up fresh vegetables (or frozen) such as mushrooms, shredded carrots, sliced cabbage, red pepper, and broccoli

2 cups of vegetable broth

1/4 cup of low sodium tamari sauce

1 tablespoon of fresh ginger, or 1/2 teaspoon of dry ginger

1/4 to 1/2 teaspoon of cayenne red pepper

2 teaspoon onion powder

2 teaspoons brown sugar or other sweetener

1/2 teaspoon garlic powder

3-4 Tablespoons of cornstarch

Heat up a nonstick skillet and then add diced onions and garlic and "dry fry" this stirring quickly to keep the onions from burning until they start to brown a little. Then add all of the cut up, prepared vegetables and continue the dry sauté, adding a little water or vegetable broth or wine to keep the mixture from sticking to the pain as needed. Water sauté this for 5-8 minutes or so.

While this is cooking cover the vegetables and let them steam a little. While the vegetables are steaming mix the vegetable broth, and all of the rest of the ingredients in a small bowl and combine them thoroughly to make a "slurry". When the vegetables are fork tender pour this sauce over the top and stir until it thickens, coating the vegetables. Serve by spooning over hot rice and top with peanuts.

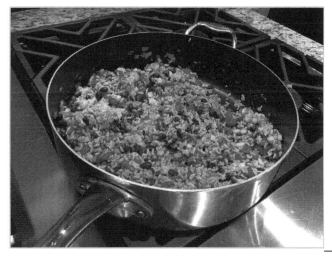

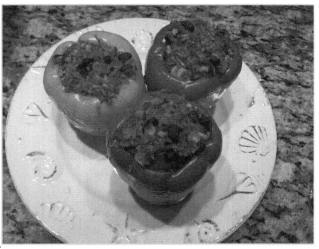

Stuffed Bell Peppers

If these are not spicy or flavorful enough, double or triple the spices to taste.

Preheat the oven to 350 degrees

Ingredients:

4 bell peppers, tops cut off, seeds removed.

1 diced onion

1 can black beans, drained and rinsed

1 cup organic frozen corn

2 cups cooked brown rice

1 14 oz can diced tomatoes

1 14 oz can tomato sauce

1 teaspoon sugar, or other sweetener like agave nectar (optional)

1 teaspoon regular or chipotle chili powder

1/2 teaspoon curry powder

1 teaspoon garlic powder

1 teaspoon onion powder

1 teaspoon low sodium tamari sauce

Method:

Place the bell peppers in a shallow baking pan or place each one into the opening of an extra large muffin pain.

Place diced onion in a dry non stick pan and sauté until soft and lightly browned, about 5 minutes.

Add the rest of the stuffing ingredients, mixing thoroughly and cooking for 8 - 10 minutes.

Place spoonfuls of the mixture into the prepared peppers. Place in the preheated oven and bake at 350 degrees for 30 minutes. Enjoy. 😊

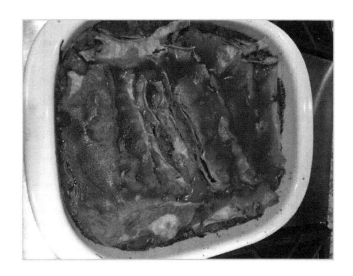

Enchilada Casserole

This casserole is not the most beautiful casserole ever made but it sure is delicious!

Ingredients:

2 cups cooked brown rice

15 oz can enchilada sauce

4 ounce can diced green Chilis

1/2 cup organic frozen corn

1/2 cup black beans, drained and rinsed

1 diced red onion

1/2 teaspoon cumin

1/2 teaspoon chili powder

1/2 teaspoon salt

1/4 teaspoon pepper

1 teaspoon garlic powder

1 teaspoon onion powder

10 Corn tortillas

1/2 bag of fresh spinach or 2 boxes of frozen, thawed and drained

1/2 cup yellow corn grits, cooked in 1 1/2 cups water

1/4 cup raw unsalted cashews

1 can of vegetarian no fat refried beans

Method:

Preheat the oven to 375 degrees

Prepare a 9 x 13 inch pan with nonstick spray or line with parchment paper.

Make the "No Cheese" Sauce:

bringing 1 1/2 cups of water with a little salt to a boil. When it begins to boil add 1/2 cup of yellow corn grits. Stir constantly and then intermittently and turn the heat down to simmer. This will be done in 5 minutes. While it finishes cooking, place the 1/4 cup of raw, unsalted cashews, 1/4 cup water, 1/4 cup nutritional yeast, 1 tsp salt, 2 tsp of onion powder 1 teaspoon of garlic powder into a Vitamix or other high speed blender. If you do not have a high speed blender then first soak the raw unsalted cashews for 2 - 4 hours and rinse and proceed with the recipe. Add the prepared corn grits and blend on high until very smooth, about 2 minutes.

Meanwhile, dry sauté the onion in a hot non stick skillet until it begins to brown. Add the spinach and just a little water and cover until the spinach wilts. Add 1/2 of the "no cheese" sauce (save the rest for pizza or something else), the rest of the spices, the black beans and the refried beans, and 1/3 of the can of enchilada sauce and heat thoroughly.

Pour another 1/3 of the can of enchilada sauce into the prepared pan.

Fill the corn tortillas with the mixture of beans and spinach, roll them up and place them seam down into the baking pan. When finished, pour the remaining 1/3 can of enchilada sauce onto the enchiladas. Bake for 30 minutes at 375 degrees. Allow to rest for 10 minutes before serving. Enjoy!

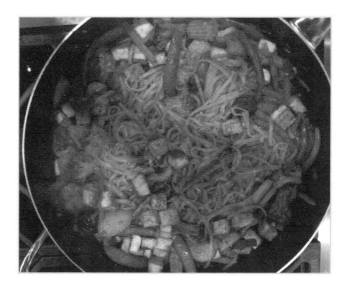

Vegan Pad Thai

Ingredients:

1 - 2 packages of brown or white rice noodles. Brown are hard to find but healthier

1 onion, diced

1 cup snow peas

1 cup sliced carrots

1 cup tofu cubes

1 bell pepper, seeded and chopped, red, yellow or orange

1 cup vegetable broth

3 teaspoons of vinegar

3 Tablespoons of natural peanut butter

the juice from 1 lemon

1 clove garlic, minced

1/2 teaspoon or more crushed red pepper

2 Tablespoons vegetarian hoisin sauce

1 teaspoon of ginger

Method:

Take the rice noodles out of the package and place in a large bowl. Cover with water and allow to soak for 1 - 4 hours.

Dry sauté the onion, garlic, and carrots in a large, deep sided non-stick skillet for about 5 minutes, until the onion is soft and translucent.

Add the rest of the vegetables and a small amount of water or vegetable broth and cover the pan while you mix up the sauce ingredients. Mix the rest of the ingredients together in a small bowl and then add to the pan, mixing with the vegetables. Drain the rice noodles and add them also to the pain and mix together well.

Desserts and Goodies

The healthiest dessert is a piece of fresh, ripe fruit or a smoothie made from fresh, ripe fruit.

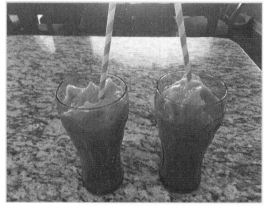

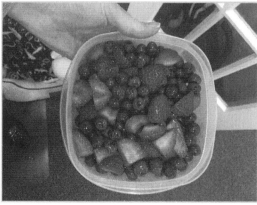

This is what you should be eating when you need to eat something sweet. This next recipe is the only healthy

335

recipe here. The rest are not horrible but they are also not exactly healthy. They are better than most of the junk people eat on a regular basis and are meant to keep you from eating real junk, but be aware that they are definitely not every day fare.

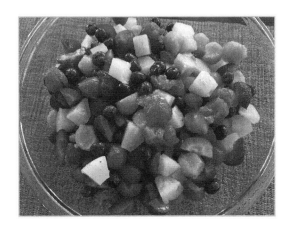

Mark's Mother's Fruit Salad Recipe

I went to college with a fellow animal lover, Mark. One day when we were studying I saw him eating this and asked him how it was made. He told me that it was his mother's recipe. This is so simple and absolutely delicious. If you bring it to a party it will be the first dish to disappear. People will eat it hand over fist. So refreshing.

Ingredients:

1 can of pineapple in natural fruit juice

2 cups fresh ripe cantaloup balls

1 cup fresh strawberries, tops cut off and sliced

1 cup fresh blueberries

2 cups watermelon balls

Method:

Place all ingredients into a large bowl. Mix thoroughly and enjoy. Refrigerate any leftovers immediately.

Again, the recipes listed here are for special occasions only, like a birthday party or a celebration. Special occasions only occur 10 - 12 times a year. It will not be easy to be skinny and fit if you eat these goodies more than occasionally. Sometimes, though, they are appropriate. Just keep them to a minimum.

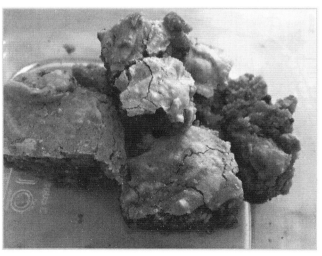

Peanut Butter and Chocolate Chip "Blondies"

Preheat the oven to 350 degrees. Prepare a 9 x 13 baking dish with non-stick spray or by lining with parchment paper.

Ingredients:

1 cup of oatmeal

1 1/2 cups of white or regular whole wheat flour

1 teaspoon cornstarch (this will soften the dough, if you prefer chewy blondies, then skip this)

1 teaspoon baking soda

1 teaspoon salt

1 cup of natural, one ingredient peanut butter

1 1/2 cups of sugar, coconut sugar, or brown sugar or a combination of these

1/2 cup of plant based milk

2 Tablespoons of flaxseed meal

2 teaspoons of vinegar

4 teaspoons of vanilla extract

1/2 cup of vegan chocolate mini chips

Method:

Place the 1 cup of oatmeal in a food processor and process until it is finely made into oat flour. Then add the whole wheat flour, cornstarch, baking soda and salt and mix thoroughly. Place this into a large mixing bowl.

Next, place the peanut butter, sugar, plant based milk, flaxseed meal, vinegar and vanilla extract into the food processor and mix thoroughly.

Gently mix the wet ingredients into the dry ingredients, being careful not to over mix or you will make the blondies tough. Add the mini chocolate chips and gently fold in. Spread this mixture evenly into the prepared pan. Place into the preheated oven and bake for 20 - 25 minutes or until a knife inserted into the center comes out clean. Do not under bake. Remove from the oven and allow to cool before cutting and removing from the pan.

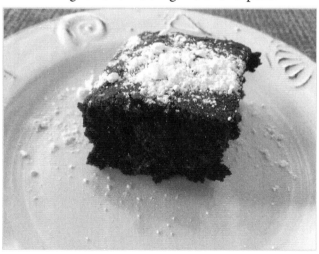

Chocolate Cake

This recipe is actually very old and was originally made during the war when there was limited access to milk and butter. It is a vegan cake but originally contained oil. I replaced the oil in this cake with applesauce and I am sure that you will find it as delicious as I do.

Preheat the oven to 350 degrees. Prepare an 8 x 8 inch baking pain with non-stick spray or by lining with parchment paper.

Ingredients:

1 1/2 cups white or regular whole wheat flour

1 cup sugar

1/3 cup cocoa powder

1/2 teaspoon salt

1 teaspoon baking soda

1/2 cup applesauce

1 Tablespoon vinegar

1 cup water or plant based milk

1 teaspoon vanilla

1/3 cup vegan chocolate mini chips

Method:

In a large bowl mix the flour, sugar, cocoa powder, salt and baking soda thoroughly. In a small bowl mix the applesauce, vinegar and water or milk and vanilla. Gently combine the wet ingredients with the dry. Then add the mini chocolate chips and pour into the prepared pan. Bake at 350 degrees for 20 to 30 minutes, or until a knife inserted into the center of the cake comes out clean.

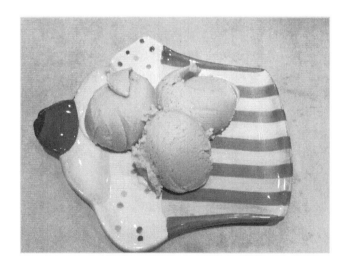

Vanilla Ice Cream

You will have to have a high speed blender and an ice cream maker for this sweet treat. Whenever you feel like you are about to break down and eat some ice cream, stop. Make this recipe and you won't need dairy ice cream any more. This stuff is just delicious, way better than any ice cream anywhere.

Ingredients:

2 cans of full fat coconut milk

1 cup of raw, unsalted cashews

1/2 to 1 cup of agave nectar or maple syrup

1 - 2 Tablespoons of vanilla extract

Method:

Place all of these ingredients into a high speed blender and blend until thoroughly combined, about 2 minutes. Start with the 1 tablespoon of vanilla and do a taste test and add up to the 2nd tablespoon of vanilla if necessary. Pour this mixture into an ice cream maker and start it up. It should be at a soft serve stage in about 1/2 an hour. Place it in a container and cover the top with waxed paper to keep it in the freezer for any amount of time. This will be quite hard when you take it out of the freezer and it will take a few minutes to become "scoopable". It is more than delicious. It is fantastic!

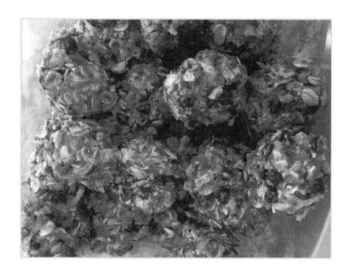

Vegan Energy Bites

These are just irresistible! I cannot believe how tasty they are. You can use them in place of granola bars for fast energy on the run. I almost always make a double batch as they are very popular and seldom last more than 2 to 3 days. They do pack a lot of calories, though, so unless you are very active, watch out!

Ingredients:

1 cup rolled oats

2/3 cup coconut flakes

1/2 cup natural, one ingredient peanut butter

1/2 cup ground flaxseed meal

1/2 cup vegan chocolate chips

1/3 cup agave nectar

1 Tablespoon chia seeds

1 teaspoon vanilla extract

1/3 cup chopped peanuts

Method:

Mix all of these ingredients together in a medium sized bowl. Cover and place into the refrigerator for at least 30 minutes. Remove from the refrigerator and scoop out by the tablespoon, forming the dough into 1 inch balls. Place into a container and store tightly covered in the refrigerator.

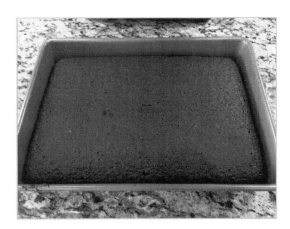

Black Bean Brownies

Preheat the oven to 350 degrees. Prepare an 8 x 8 baking pan for thick brownies or a 9 x 13 pan for thinner brownies by spraying with non-stick spray or lining with parchment paper.

Ingredients:

1 1/2 cups of white or regular whole wheat flour

1 1/2 cups sugar

1 1/4 cups cocoa powder

1 Tablespoon instant coffee powder

1 teaspoon baking powder

1/2 teaspoon salt

1 15 ounce can of black beans, rinsed and drained

1 teaspoon vanilla

2 cups of water or plant based milk

1/2 cup of walnuts, pecans or vegan chocolate chips

Method:

Combine the flour, sugar, cocoa powder, instant coffee, baking powder and salt in a large bowl. Mix thoroughly.

Place the drained and rinsed black beans, vanilla and water or milk into a food processor and combine throughly.

Add the bean mixture to the dry ingredients, mixing until throughly combined but avoid over mixing. Spread this mixture into the prepared baking pan and place in the oven for 20 - 30 minutes, rotating the pan halfway through the baking process. Bake at 350 degrees until a knife inserted into the center of the brownies comes out clean. The smaller pan will take a little longer than the larger pan as the brownies will be thicker.

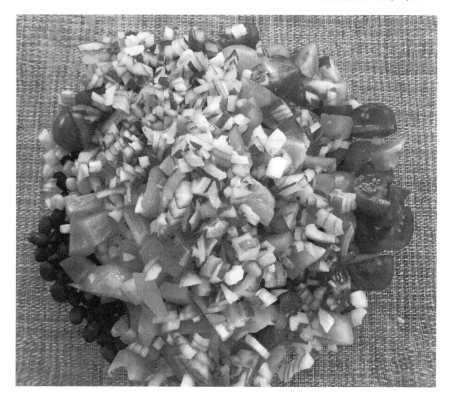

Chapter 8 Sample Plan

Here is a one week sample plan of a menu to eat and an exercise plan to follow for those of you who like it written out. I am making this really easy because it IS really easy. All it requires is that you stick to the plan most of the time. Life is complicated. There is no way that you will be able to do this all of the time, but all that is required is that you do it most of the time. Remember, you can buy two bananas for a dollar in many convenience stores. Stick to the plan!

Prep Day: I will assume this is a Sunday, but you know your schedule better than I do. On prep day, make a big pot of soup. Maybe even 2 pots of soup. There should be A LOT of soup. Eat some of the soup for lunch, maybe even supper and put the rest into large serving size containers. Put one in the fridge for work the next day and put the others in the freezer.

Also make the "No Cheesy" Sprinkle. Put half of it in an airtight container to leave at home and the other half in an airtight container to take to work to put on your salad along with some fat free dressing.

Make yourself some low sugar freezer jam as well. Then it will be on hand when you need it.

Every day you should make a pitcher of green tea or hibiscus tea so it will available for you to drink. Add a little sugar to it if you need to, but gradually reduce the amount of sugar in the tea until you can drink it without sugar.

Day One: (Monday)

Breakfast: Whole Grain Hot Cereal, 1 1/2 cups prepared, 1/2 cup of plant based milk on the cereal and 2 - 3 pieces of fresh whole fruit. You can put a little bit of sugar on the cereal if you need to. Add cinnamon if you like. Do not add any fat.

On the way out the door grab your container of soup and make yourself a quick fresh garden salad with romaine lettuce, bell peppers, cucumbers, tomatoes, etc. Bring a bottle of fat free dressing to work with you and place it in the refrigerator at work or leave it in a lunch cooler. Bring a few pieces of fruit as well, just to hold you over if you are still hungry or if you need a snack. If you are pressed for time in the morning, make the salad the night before so it is ready to go.

Lunch: It's soup and salad time. Heat up your soup. While it heats up, eat your salad. When you finish the soup if you are still hungry, have a piece of fresh fruit or two or three.

Supper: Sweet potatoes and some steamed broccoli. When you get home from work, poke several holes into 2 - 4 sweet potatoes and put them on a foil lined baking pan. Bake at 375 for 1 to 1 and a half hours. While they bake, you are going to do your workout so change your clothes!

Monday workout: 30 minutes of cardio or aerobic exercise. You want to sweat, that is the point. Walk up and down the stairs over and over if it is cold and yucky outside, or use a treadmill, or go for a walk or run outside if the weather permits. You should be able to talk but not sing for 30 minutes and there should be some perspiration involved. Then do 20 minutes of strengthening exercises, such as pushups, sit-ups, planks, squats, bicep curls, super mans, etc. Just keep working until you have finished 20 minutes. Then for the last 10 minutes, stretch all of your muscle groups. Now, hit the shower and when you are finished with the shower, your sweet potatoes will be cooked, Throw a bag of frozen broccoli in the microwave, or steam 2 - 3 cups of the fresh stuff in a saucepan with a little water until they are fork tender and there is your supper. Add a little brown sugar and / or cinnamon to top the sweet potatoes if you need to. Add a little "no cheesy" sprinkle and some salt and pepper to top the broccoli if you need to. After supper, if you are still hungry, have a piece of fruit or two or three and then get out of the kitchen and go do something else. Day one, is DONE!

Day Two: (Tuesday)

Breakfast: Same as Monday. If you eat the same breakfast you don't have much to think about. Just get it done. Whole Grain Hot Cereal, 1 1/2 cups prepared, 1/2 cup of plant based milk on the cereal and 2 - 3 pieces of fresh whole fruit. You can put a little bit of sugar on the cereal if you need to. Add cinnamon if you like. Do not add any fat.

Lunch: Did you have any sweet potatoes or broccoli left over from last night? If you did then that is your lunch today. If you didn't, make yourself a peanut butter and jelly sandwich with whole grain bread, homemade low sugar strawberry jam and one ingredient peanut butter. If you have a big appetite make two sandwiches. Bring 2 -3 pieces of fresh whole fruit as well.

Supper: Burger and Fries. See the recipe section and make some bean burgers and bake up some regular or sweet potato fries. While the fries are baking, do 15 to 20 minutes of cardio exercise or some strength training.

After supper if you are still hungry eat some fresh whole fruit. Then get out of the kitchen and go do something else.

Day three (Wednesday)

Breakfast: Once again, keep it simple. The important thing is that you are full. Stay full so when people come to work with a bunch of junk you won't be tempted to eat it. Whole Grain Hot Cereal, 1 1/2 cups prepared, 1/2 cup of plant based milk on the cereal and 2 - 3 pieces of fresh whole fruit. You can put a little bit of sugar on the cereal if you need to. Add cinnamon if you like. Do not add any fat. Or have a piece of whole grain toast! Just make sure you eat something!

Lunch: Make another salad, grab another tub of frozen soup and out the door you go. You are getting this done!

Wednesday workout: Again, do 30 minutes of cardio or aerobic exercise. You want to sweat, that is the point. Walk up and down the stairs over and over if it is cold and yucky outside, or use a treadmill, or go for a walk or run outside if the weather permits. You should be able to talk but not sing for 30 minutes and there should be some perspiration involved. Then do 20 minutes of strengthening exercises, such as pushups, sit-ups, planks, squats, bicep curls, super mans, etc. Just keep working until you have finished 20 minutes. Then for the last 10 minutes, stretch all of your muscle groups. You can use video exercise programs if you like, the important part is you get it done!

Supper on Wednesday: Make fajitas. (See recipe section)

Day four (Thursday)

Breakfast: This is my go to breakfast. If you have another similar one, then do it. The important part is that you are full. This is done to avoid the load of junk food options that are waiting everywhere to sabotage your efforts. Whole Grain Hot Cereal, 1 1/2 cups prepared, 1/2 cup of plant based milk on the cereal and 2 - 3 pieces of fresh whole fruit. You can put a little bit of sugar on the cereal if you need to. Add cinnamon if you like. Do not add any fat.

Lunch: leftover fajitas if you had any left, if not grab a container of soup and some pieces of fresh fruit as you run out the door.

Supper: Taco Salad (See recipe section)

Workout: 30 minutes of cardio, 20 minutes of strength training and 10 minutes of stretching. You've got this!

Day five (Friday)

Breakfast: Last day of the week! Once again, keeping it simple. The important thing is that you are full. Stay full! Don't slip up! Whole Grain Hot Cereal, 1 1/2 cups prepared, 1/2 cup of plant based milk on the cereal and 2 - 3 pieces of fresh whole fruit. You can put a little bit of sugar on the cereal if you need to. Add cinnamon if you like. Do not add any fat.

Lunch: Fast Food restaurant. Get a smoothie, salad or vegan sandwich or make your own at home. Or, eat your soup, salad and fruit. It's almost time for the weekend! You are DOING this!

Supper: You have a choice. If Friday night is your out to dinner night, then go out. Order the healthiest thing you can find on the menu, like a big salad with no cheese or meat and the dressing on the side or a veggie burger with a side salad. This will be your slight "cheat" meal of the week. Enjoy yourself with the awesome company you are in. The food will be "okay" but the highlight of the evening is going to be your awesome friends and or family members. This is what life is about, loving the beautiful people you are blessed to have in your life. If you are not a Friday night out kind of a person, then it will be pizza night. Make a fresh,

353

homemade pizza using the recipe in this book. If you have time to make the pizza crust that is great, if not, make sure that you buy a whole wheat already prepared crust with no more than 20 percent of the calories coming from added fat. Also make sure that there is no cheese added to the crust already. I swear, they try to hide cheese everywhere! Heat the oven to 425, prepare a pan with parchment paper, make the "no cheese" sauce(see recipe section for the pizza recipe) and then spread the pizza crust with the no cheese sauce, then the marinara sauce and then the cut up vegetables, onions, olives, spinach, etc.

No workout on Friday, unless you are super hard core. Take a rest day!

Saturday Morning: Time for a run! A serious, long run, or swim, or bike, or whatever it is that you like. Run a few miles. If running is your thing, run 6 - 8 miles, then stretch out. If running is not yet your thing, run or walk 2 - 3 miles, then stretch out. Take the dog or another family member and have a great time. Run fast enough that it is a little annoying but not so fast that you can't talk. When you get back home, mix up a batch of "no muffin top muffins" and pop them in the oven while you go take a shower. When they are finished baking you will be done with your shower and can enjoy your breakfast.

Lunch on Saturday: Check out a pho noodle soup restaurant in your area. Most of them have vegetarian pho noodle soup. Yummy.

Supper on Saturday: Make a veggie lasagna (see recipe section). This will be big enough to eat for a few meals if your family is small. Serve this with a side salad and some whole wheat french bread if you like.

Sunday is FUNday! Time for waffles or pancakes. (See recipe section) Enjoy your delicious breakfast. Some people like to try to make a tofu scramble. It is not my thing, but the recipes are widely available online. Hashed brown potatoes are also pretty easy and pretty delicious (see recipe section).

Lunch on Sunday: Time to make another big pot of soup or chili and prepare for the upcoming week. Have soup or chili for lunch and supper. No workout on Sunday unless you are really hardcore. It is a rest day.

Week one is in the bag! Congratulations! For the next week you just keep this up. Whole grains and fruit for breakfast, soup, salad or sandwiches for lunch, a mildly ornate supper. Please see my fellow low fat vegan recipe makers like the Brand New Vegan, Potatostrong, the Vegan 8, and Forks over Knives for all kinds of delicious recipes and ideas for supper. I try to keep weekday breakfasts and lunch pretty simple. The important thing is that you have a plan. Remember, a failure to plan is a plan to fail! Don't let this happen! Be prepared. Don't let yourself get desperate. You can do this!!!! We can all do this!!!!

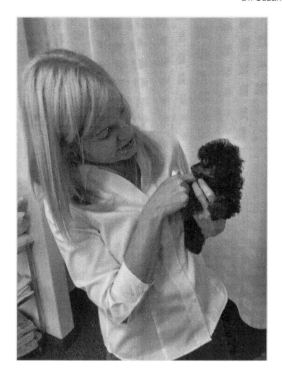

About the Author

Dr. Suzanne Foxx is a physical therapist in private practice in Newport News, Virginia. She has a special interest in nutrition and exercise and the ability of the body to heal itself given the right circumstances. She graduated from Christopher Newport University and Old Dominion University and is married to her high school sweetheart. They have two grown sons. She enjoys running, reading, aquariums and playing with her poodles in her spare time.

Skinny & Fit but Never Hungry a Bit

Suggestions For Further information

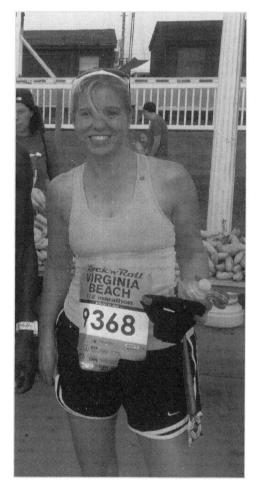

I have read each of these books and found them very helpful:

"Eat to Live" by Dr. Joel Fuhrman

"Eat and Run" by Scott Jurek

"Disease Proof Your Children" by Dr. Joel Fuhrman

"Salt, Sugar and Fat" by Michael Moss

"The Engine 2 Diet" by Rip Esselstyn

"PlantStrong" by Rip Esselstyn

"Prevent and Reverse Heart Disease" by Dr. Caldwell Esselstyn

"Veganist" by Kathy Freston

"The Starch Solution" by Dr. John McDougall

"The China Study" by Dr. T. Colin Cambell

"Finding Ultra" by Rich Roll

"The Mad Cowboy" by Howard Lyman

"Proteinaholic" by Dr. Garth Davis

"The Pleasure Trap" by Dr. Alan Goldhammer and Dr. Doug Lisle

"Dr. Neal Barnard's Program for Reversing Diabetes" by Dr. Neal Barnard

"How Not to Die" by Dr. Michael Gregor

There are several wonderful documentaries out now, most notably Forks over Knives, Eating You Alive and Plant

Pure Nation. They are all wonderful and very helpful in living a plant based, oil free life.

Dr. John McDougall has many resources available on Youtube. I, myself, have a YouTube Channel called Skinny and Fit TV. Many of the other authors above have lectures available for free on YouTube. On Facebook I have found "The Brand New Vegan", the Vegan8, Forks over Knives, the No Meat Athlete and "Potatostrong" to be particularly helpful for finding delicious, healthy and easy recipes. There are many, many very good resources available for eating and living a plant based, vegan, no oil added diet. You can even order frozen, ready to eat whole food plant based meals delivered right to your door from "Plant Pure Nation". I wish you the best on your journey and don't be a stranger! Let me know if I have helped. Here's to plants for the win every time!